Ageing Societies

Ageing Societies:

A Comparative Introduction

Virpi Timonen

 Open University Press

Open University Press
McGraw-Hill Education
McGraw-Hill House
Shoppenhangers Road
Maidenhead
Berkshire
England
SL6 2QL

email: enquiries@openup.co.uk
world wide web: www.openup.co.uk

and Two Penn Plaza, New York, NY 10121–2289, USA

First published 2008
Copyright © Virpi Timonen 2008

A catalogue record of this book is available from the British Library

ISBN–10: 0-335-22269-2 (pb)   0-335-22270-6 (hb)
ISBN–13: 978-0-335-22269-8 (pb)   978-0-335-22270-4 (hb)

Library of Congress Cataloguing-in-Publication Data
CIP data applied for

Typeset by YHT Ltd, London
Printed in the UK by Bell and Bain Ltd, Glasgow

The *McGraw·Hill* Companies

Contents

List of figures, tables and boxes

List of figures

List of tables

List of boxes

Preface

This book aims to provide an *intelligent introduction* to some of the key dimensions of the complex phenomenon known as 'ageing'. The word *introduction* implies that many different aspects of ageing are flagged and discussed briefly: the intention is to cover a lot of ground without specializing in any one aspect of ageing. Inevitably, this means that the subtlety and detail of many questions and debates is not fully explored; this is, however, inevitable in view of the intention to provide readers with a good overview of the topic within the confines of a single book. While the general approach is international and comparative in that no single country or group of countries is the exclusive or predominant focus, the book does not pretend to be genuinely global in its scope. In particular, ageing in the developing world is discussed only in very general terms. The word *intelligent* indicates that the book seeks to crystallize a lot of information and to highlight the interconnections between the health, economic and social aspects of ageing, and hopes to accomplish this in a way that is neither patronizing nor intimidating.

Following the first chapter that makes the case for the importance of studying and understanding ageing, Chapter 2 gives a brief outline of the dynamics of population ageing ('demography 101'). From this demographic background, we proceed to analysing in Chapter 3 the changing family and social contexts of ageing: the importance of social engagement for happy and healthy ageing, whether it is achieved through family networks or wider 'personal communities' is stressed here. It is not possible to engage with debates about the implications of ageing without understanding the changing health status of ageing populations, and Chapter 4 provides the readers with a discussion of the dynamics of health in older populations. Incomes in old age are another key area, and Chapter 5 discusses the shifting balance between pensions and employment as sources of income in older age. Chapter 6 seeks to provide a balanced and dispassionate view on the thorny issue of 'affordability' of ageing and outlines the strategies that governments have adopted in reaction to the real and perceived challenges brought about by ageing. Chapter 7 broaches the complex area of long term care for older people, with a focus on clearly outlining the differences and overlaps between informal and formal care, and the roles of public and private actors in providing and financing care. Chapter 8 deepens the care theme by discussing different types and locations of care, with an emphasis on home and community care, which are argued to be the predominant preference of individuals and, increasingly, policymakers. Chapter 9 discusses ageism and the impact of older people as voters, consumers and individuals who may not want to conform to the stereotypes associated with 'elderly people'. Chapter 10 concludes by arguing that societies and individuals are only now beginning to adjust to ageing, and that major changes in the way we view older people are both necessary and desirable.

As is evident from the above description of chapter contents, the book covers many of the factors that exert an influence *on* and in turn are influenced *by* population ageing: families, lifestyles, work, retirement, health and care. One of the key messages of this book lies in the fact that almost everything that we study in the area of ageing is both a *de*pendent and an *in*dependent variable: family change, for instance, is both affected by ageing (longer co-existence of older and younger generations gives greater scope for relationship building across generations) and affects the process ageing (smaller family size feeds into population ageing). The fascination of ageing as an area of investigation lies in its multidimensionality and the many connections between these dimensions. This characteristic is also, unfortunately, the biggest stumbling block for newcomers to the study of ageing: it seems to cover such a wide array of subtopics that making sense of them all, let alone seeing the links between them, can appear to be an impossible challenge. This book hopes to show that the 'health' and 'economic' aspects of ageing are influenced by the 'social' aspects of ageing, and vice versa. As such, ageing is one of the most rewarding topics of inter-disciplinary research, and arguably can and should be approached from the multiple angles that this book seeks to briefly flag. This inter-dependence of different aspects of ageing also constitutes effective ammunition against the argument that ageing inevitably leads to negative consequences for economies and societies. The way in which societies and policies are organized profoundly shapes the impact of ageing. Whether ageing is (and is seen as) problematic is entirely a social and political decision: there is nothing inevitably deleterious about ageing.

The book therefore seeks to convince the readers of the overwhelming importance of *policies* in shaping the individual experiences and societal impacts of ageing. In this respect, the book hopes to contribute to the realization that many of the impacts of ageing that are commonly portrayed as inevitable are in fact eminently malleable by political decisions: politics and policy really matter in determining the effects of ageing on societies and individuals. While ageing is evidently a biological process (albeit a still poorly understood one), it is also a social phenomenon. As such it is one that we all, young and old, influence in important ways. This book hopes to convince the readers that ageing is not boring, threatening or depressing, that it has enormous relevance for the young and the old alike, and that, above all, it is a great human achievement that most societies and individuals are only just beginning to understand, adjust to and cherish.

Acknowledgements

Enormous thanks are due to four people who have made a real difference – to some extent to the content, and certainly to the feasibility – of this book (in the order of their appearance in my life):

My mother, Liisa, who during our sojourn in Australia (where this book was completed) looked after the girls (during a leave from work enabled by the Finnish state) and thereby freed me up to write at a faster pace than would otherwise have been possible. She can testify to the argument that inter-generational transfers flow predominantly from the older to the younger generations ... *Kiitos Äiti.*

My husband, Iain, whose patient deciphering of my illegible manuscript and skilful typing ... or rather whose constant humour, support, resource-fulness, commitment and unfailing (if misguided) admiration of my work have been an enormous boost to me for over a decade.

My daughters Suvi and Anja who, despite being absolutely insufferable at times, are the best girls in the whole world – by some distance. I hope they will sustain their amazing *panache, joie de vivre* and sheer determination (sisu!) for many, many decades to come, and always remain great friends and support for each other all the way into their old age ... sometime in the early twenty-second century ...

Thanks of a somewhat lesser but still considerable magnitude are due to several other people. They are too numerous to list individually, and I can only highlight some here. Rachel Gear, Senior Commissioning Editor at McGraw-Hill, encouraged me by liking the idea of this book back in early 2004, and by applying sympathy and subtle pressure at just the right times. Robbie Gilligan has been a great enabler in my academic life since I entered Trinity College Dublin, helping me to do the things that I want to do in ageing research. I have been extremely lucky to work with several highly intelligent, motivated and good humoured people in SPARC: Martha, Ciara, Colette and Ana – you are simply brilliant, and so much appreciated as col-leagues. Of course, my association and work with these and other valued colleagues in SPARC would not have been possible without the vision of a certain modest Hibernophile ... for which we are all deeply grateful. Trinity colleagues from disciplines as diverse as medical gerontology, demography and economics have helped me to better understand the diversity of ageing research, and given me wonderful opportunities to participate in inter-disciplinary work. The students who have taken my social policy and ageing course (and perhaps especially the ones who gave critical feedback) also deserve some credit for forcing me to clarify my thinking and improve my presentation. In Canberra, a *fantastic* place that is forever in my heart, several people looked after me during the last stages of the writing of this book both in terms of office space and entertainment: special thanks are due to Simon Bronitt and other staff at the National Europe Centre of the Australian National University, Jenny and Rodney Berrill whose beautiful house bordering on the bush we occupied for a blissful four months, and Andrea Gleason and Ben Reilly, great friends. Many other colleagues and friends are extremely helpful in sustaining and broadening my interests within and outside the field of ageing, and provide amusing diversions to various avenues in life – let's just say that they know who they are, and where those avenues led up to … Ding Dong Dang: I'll be back when I turn 80. That's a promise.

PART ONE
SOCIAL CONTEXTS OF AGEING

1 The importance of understanding ageing

Introduction

This chapter highlights the nature of ageing as an individual and societal experience and makes the case for the importance of analysing ageing from a number of different perspectives. Ageing is a phenomenon that affects everyone, not only the older population. While ageing is currently most manifest and has given rise to much discussion and many (attempted) policy changes in the developed countries, ageing is also a truly global phenomenon that is proceeding at a very fast pace in many parts of the developing world. Despite the fact that ageing is becoming an increasingly widespread experience, age related policies, practices and consequently the actual lived experience of ageing differ greatly between countries and regions of the world. The chapter outlines the main theoretical frameworks that have been developed to explain the way societies treat older people. The chapter also contains a brief introduction to the complex issue of attitudes towards ageing which have a powerful influence on the ways we understand, study and experience ageing. We will return to the topic of attitudes towards ageing in the last two chapters of the book.

What is ageing?

'Ageing' is a term that occurs increasingly frequently in the media, in political debates and in conversations, yet the meaning of this term is rarely spelled out. Even after we have defined ageing, we may be uncertain of the rationale for *studying* ageing. Young adults in particular can find the study of 'ageing' and 'older people' irrelevant or even off putting. This attitude is brought about by lack of appreciation of the fact that ageing is one of the most important global phenomena at present. In the developed world virtually everybody who is 'young' today can confidently expect to become 'old' in the future. This is a major change from the past when higher death rates across the age spectrum meant that many did not survive past early childhood or through other hazardous periods and events (such as famines, epidemics or, even more commonplace, childbirth in the case of women). While a lamentably large proportion of the populations of developing countries still does not survive into old age, in virtually all countries and regions of the world increasing proportions of the population do reach the age at which they are considered 'old'. One of the many surprising facts about ageing is that already, some two-thirds of the world's older people (defined as those aged 60 or older) reside in developing countries. Ageing is a truly global phenomenon.

Young people are affected by ageing to a much greater extent than they often appreciate or want to admit. Responding to the above argument on the universal experience of 'ageing', a younger person may retort that while they are admittedly 'ageing' they have certainly not yet reached (and will not for a long time reach) 'old age'. While this distinction is perfectly sound, it still masks the important inter-linkages between 'ageing' and 'growing old'. Most importantly, 'young people' are affected (without usually realizing it) by the simple fact that, with survival into old age having become a common experience, people have come to *expect* long lifespans: whereas in the past few individuals survived into old age, virtually everyone in the developed world can now proceed in the fairly safe knowledge that they will survive to 65 (or whatever the perceived threshold of old age is in their respective country) and beyond. Human life is overshadowed by death to an indescribably lesser degree than it was in the past: indeed at present it is possible in the rich world to survive to the age of 40 or even beyond without experiencing the death of any close relatives – whereas this was extremely rare in the not too distant past. This does not mean, of course, that everybody always makes decisions in accordance with this expectation, or behaves in a way that would be 'rational' in view of the realistic expectation of a long life! Indeed, it is arguable that while increasingly widespread, the experience of ageing is still (historically speaking) so novel to human beings that we have not had time to adapt to it. We will return to this topic of necessary and desirable modifications in behaviours and policies in several of the subsequent chapters.

We will now proceed to addressing two questions that are fundamental to the structure and purpose of the book, and indeed to the study of ageing on the whole:

- What is ageing?
- Why is ageing important, and why do we need to understand it better?

Despite the great significance of ageing, its meaning and causes remain unknown to most people. In answering the first question posed above ('What is ageing?') it is helpful to examine ageing from three different angles, namely (1) individual ageing; (2) population ageing; and (3) qualitative changes in ageing (OECD 1996).

Box 1.1   Three different aspects of ageing

Individual ageing: people living longer.

Population ageing: a greater number of older people in relation to
                                      younger people within a population group.

Qualitative aspects of ageing: different patterns of activity, changing expectations.

Source: OECD (1996).

We can view ageing at the level of individuals where it consists of people on average living longer than members of earlier generations (*individual ageing*). The survival of most people into increasingly older age is historically a very recent development, and one that was in most countries started by a decline in the rate at which babies and children were dying at an early age. It was not uncommon, until a rather short time ago, for many babies to perish in early infanthood due to infectious diseases and poor nutrition. Better hygiene practices, availability of medicines and vaccines, and better and cleaner food and water served to bring about huge declines in infant mortality, first in the richer world and subsequently (although still regrettably slowly in some cases) in poorer countries. This decline in infant and childhood mortality was complemented by declines in mortality at older ages, and as a combined result of these reductions in childhood and adulthood mortality increasing numbers of people reach the age at which they are considered to be 'old'. For instance, whereas the average person born around 1570 in England could expect to live for approximately 40 years (Wrigley and Schofield 1989), nowadays boys and girls born in the UK could expect on average to live to 76.6 years and 81.0 years of age respectively (National Statistics UK 2007).

Following, and in some cases in parallel with, declining mortality that manifests itself in more people living into older age, people have adopted different fertility behaviours. To put it simply, people are having fewer babies than they used to, due to the availability of and desire to use contraceptive devices, increased preference for paid employment and leisure over childrearing, and also the realistic assumption that any children they have will survive (not a rational expectation in the past when infant mortality rates were higher and it was 'rational' to have many children in order to ensure that at least some survived to contribute to the household economy and to provide care and security to ageing parents). When combined with reduced and in many cases still declining birth rates, individual ageing translates into an increase in the *share* of older people in the population as a whole (*population ageing*).

In summary, population ageing is driven by the so-called demographic transition, which consists of a shift from *high fertility* and *high mortality* to *low(er) fertility* and *low(er) mortality* rates. Whereas in the past older people accounted only for a very small proportion of the overall population, their share has now surpassed 20 percent and is soon set to surpass 25 percent of the total population in many countries. This is sometimes referred to as 'greying of the population'.

Box 1.2   The demographic transition

High fertility and *high* mortality

towards

Low fertility and *low* mortality

Chapter 2 explains the processes behind population ageing in greater detail, and also provides further data on population ageing in different parts of the world. For now it is sufficient to note that, with few exceptions, the populations of virtually all countries in the world are ageing, meaning that the (numerical) balance between younger and older people is shifting in favour of the older age groups.

The third, least well understood and most controversial, aspect of ageing consists of the *qualitative changes* that are occurring in people's lives as they live longer. The behaviours and characteristics that are expected from, and associated with, older people are constantly evolving. Whereas in the past many people might have considered it inappropriate that older people pay a lot of attention to their personal well being and appearance, such behaviours have become generally more accepted, and even expected. In many countries, the demands are increasing that people remain in paid employment for longer than has been the case in recent decades. In political rhetoric, policy documents and advertising these changes in older people's activities and behaviour are sometimes labeled and portrayed as 'active' or 'positive' ageing. We will return to these themes in Chapters 9 and 10.

Why study ageing?

We have already highlighted a number of reasons why understanding ageing is important. Adapting an outline by the United Nations (2002), the following list summarizes the key rationales for studying ageing:

1   Ageing is a *pervasive* phenomenon in that it affects everyone, not only the older parts of the population, and *global* in that it affects all

regions of the world. As a result, ageing has important implications for inter-generational, intra-generational and also international equity (see Chapters 3, 5 and 6).

2   Ageing has *significant consequences* for the economy, the society and politics. In the economic sphere, for instance, ageing (together with policies and practices that influence the behaviour of older people) can affect savings and investments, consumption patterns, labour markets, public expenditure, taxation and income transfers between generations. Note that while the impacts of ageing are undoubtedly significant, the nature of the impact does not have to be negative. For instance, an ageing population does not inevitably lead to a sluggish economy.

3   Ageing of the magnitude that we are witnessing today is an *unprecedented* phenomenon, and as such offers plenty of new material to study. Ageing is very likely to be *enduring* and *irreversible*. We are unlikely to return to a situation where people are dying earlier and having more children. Ageing is also an ongoing phenomenon, the limits of which are not yet known. We still know very little about most aspects of ageing and as the impacts and implications of ageing are constantly evolving, there is a need to adapt our thinking in line with this evolution.

In short, ageing is both *universal* and *diverse*. While ageing impacts on everyone and (virtually) everything in society, politics and the economy, its impact differs greatly by country and by policy area. It is also easy to exaggerate the implications of ageing; this book hopes to show that age often overlaps and interacts with other important factors such as gender and social class that are, together with ageing, responsible for producing inequalities and other socially significant outcomes. While individuals and governments should respond to ageing by modifying policies and attitudes, the nature and extent of these responses can be counter-productive or misguided (Chapter 6).

We will now turn to a brief discussion of definitions of old age, followed by a discussion of the need to redefine old age, and the main theoretical frameworks that researchers have developed in trying to understand ageing and its societal roots and impacts.

Defining 'old age'

While defining 'ageing' is quite straightforward and population ageing can in fact be presented in a mathematical formula where the proportions between the strictly age delineated 'younger' and 'older' population groups are shifting, the task of defining 'old age' is considerably more complex and inevitably involves venturing into the less clear cut territory of social constructions, attitudes and even values. For the purposes of most comparative statistics, old age begins at 60 or 65. Little reflection is needed to realize that this is a rather arbitrary definition. First, as Chapters 2 and 4 will point out, life expectancies vary greatly between different parts of the world and between different socioeconomic groups within countries (not to mention the significant difference in male and female life expectancies in many countries). Whereas only a relatively small proportion of the population of a very poor country survives beyond the age of 65 ('becomes old'), some demographers now predict that as many as one in three female children born today in some of the world's richest countries will reach the age of 100. In the light of increased life expectancies and dramatic differences in life expectancies and the quality of life of the older people both within countries and between different parts of the world, it is obvious that the conventional (age-based) definition of 'old age' is inadequate and even misleading.

There are many different ways of defining age (Cavanaugh and Whitbourne 1999). *Chronological age* is the most straightforward, but also in many ways the least informative, indicator of age: it simply refers to the number of years someone has lived. *Biological age* refers to the functioning of the body and its component parts (such as the cardiovascular system). People's bodies age (senesce) at different rates, determined by a complex mix of external and internal factors. While longevity is influenced by one's genetic make-up, other factors can override the benefit of 'longevity genes': a person who has not had the benefit of a nutritious diet, clean air and water, exercise and good medical care is likely to age considerably faster (and to die sooner) than someone who has been able and willing to 'invest' in their health. *Psychological age* refers to an individual's memory, intelligence, feelings and motivation: someone who is convinced that they are unfit and incapable of participating in many activities can often appear much older than a person of similar chronological and biological age who believes that 'old age' is not an impediment to them.

However, perhaps the most influential among different definitions of age is the *sociocultural age* that is attached to a person. This refers to society's expectations of older people. Regardless of how older people view their bodies, minds and capabilities, society can place extensive limits on their ability to act in accordance with those views. All societies tend to assign older people certain 'age appropriate' roles, such as retirement and grandparenthood, and 'suitable' patterns of activity or inactivity, such as gardening, bingo, bus tours or retirement from paid work. These expectations and attitudes, and the extent to which they are at variance with older people's own attitudes and aspirations, are the topic of Chapters 9 and 10.

In summary, it is crucial to understand that there is no one correct or straightforward definition of 'old age'. All definitions are incomplete, and the most common ones are often arbitrary. Most attributes of old age are culturally determined. Unfortunately, we have no equivalent of the sex/ gender distinction developed by feminist scholars to differentiate between the biological and socially assigned ages.

The increasing numbers of older people and changing patterns of activity among them have led us to reflect on the adjustments that should be made to the way we think about ageing. A number of chapters in this book examine various aspects of the societal and attitudinal changes that are accompanying, or arguably should accompany, population ageing. Chapter 3 refers to changing roles of older people in families and other social contexts; Chapter 5 explores the established and gradually changing expectations around work and retirement; Chapter 6 discusses the role of attitudes, expectations and commonly used definitions in creating the perception that ageing is unaffordable; Chapters 7 and 8 refer to the ways in which our assumptions about older people's needs and wishes govern the organization of long term care; and Chapters 9 and 10 outline the ways in which the political, social and consumer behaviours of older people are both a reflection of their own and society's changing attitudes towards ageing.

Theories of ageing

The field of ageing studies (or gerontology as it is sometimes called) is not particularly theory laden (or theory rich, depending on your fondness for theories). This has both positive and negative implications. On the positive side, students of ageing can operate largely free from the constraints of overarching theories and as a result are perhaps more inclined to collect and analyse a rich variety of data in the absence of any preconceived notions of what 'the reality' should look like. For the same reason, they are also free to formulate new theories and explanatory frameworks, which is always an exciting enterprise. On the negative side, the absence of widely utilized theoretical frameworks can make the study of ageing somewhat unwieldy and dissatisfying for the more theoretically minded individuals, particularly those who are keen to test theory driven hypotheses. For some, this paucity of theories means that the study of various aspects of ageing, or gerontology, is not a fully fledged academic discipline. While a number of 'theories' of ageing are outlined below, this is done in comfortable recognition of the fact that these may not in all respects fulfil all of the demanding criteria for a 'theory' and are perhaps better described as explanatory frameworks that seek to make sense of the social processes related to ageing. This section also omits to describe several other 'theories' of ageing as they are deemed to fall far short of the definition of a theory and were developed primarily for descriptive (rather than explanatory) and prescriptive (advocating a 'better' perspective on older people) purposes.

The broad sociological school of thought known as structural function-alism has spawned many of the theories promulgated, applied and tested by those researching different aspects of later life. Functionalist approaches such as the disengagement and modernization theories have focused on social structures and institutions and primarily strive to unearth the functions that these social arrangements serve or seek to fulfil, and the norms and values that contribute to the maintenance of order in societies. According to the *disengagement theory* ageing leads to an exit from many roles and duties at the societal, individual and psychological levels (Cumming and Henry 1961). Disengagement theory implies that older adults who recognize the need to disengage for the good of the society are able to age 'successfully': disen-gagement from society is good for older people and good for society. Com-mon good and goals of efficiency and fairness are served when younger people take over demanding and influential positions and roles from older people, who in turn can narrow their spheres of activity to more manageable levels in preparation for physical and mental decline and ultimately death. Retirement and widowhood have in many societies come to be seen as the main 'rites of passage' into old age: retirement from (paid) work constitutes an exit from the active breadwinner role adopted by most men, and widow-hood can be seen as similarly involving a woman's exit from her role of serving and supporting her husband. According to disengagement theory, society prescribes the roles that are appropriate for older people, and the majority of older people more or less willingly 'slot into' these roles.

Disengagement theory is a rather ambitious attempt to generalize societal expectations and behavioural patterns associated with old age across different cultures and over time. The basic premise of this theory is functionalist: it argues that all societies need to deal with and prepare for the certain event of death and the slightly less certain but still widespread phenomena of illness and disability in old age. The starting point of the theory is therefore 'morbid' in that it focuses on the individual and societal needs generated by the inevitability of loss of function, disease and death. The main criticism levelled against this theory is that its search for a universal pattern of disengagement generalizes too much, and also paints a picture of older people as passive actors who have very low expectations of old age. There is nothing inevitable or 'functionally necessary' about people leaving employment at the age of 65 or adopting other passive roles. Variation in the experience of ageing across time and different countries, and the dramatically changing patterns of activity among older people in many parts of the world demonstrate that there is no universal pattern of ageing characterized by disengagement and passivity. While it is undeniable that many features of current policies and practices (such as compulsory retirement) could be construed as supporting evidence for this theory, it is also increasingly evident that societies are trying to devise ways of continuing the engagement of older people in the economic and social spheres of life (the most obvious example is the attempted extension of working lives into older ages). The 'activity theory' of ageing was developed to counter many of the assumptions and arguments associated with the disengagement theory: the 'activity theory' is, however, conceptually rather weak and is essentially prescriptive and almost 'ideological' in nature as its primary aim was arguably to highlight 'positive' aspects of ageing.

The *modernization theory* (Cowgill and Holmes 1972) argues that the status of older people is inversely related to the level of industrialization. In pre-industrial societies older people had control of scarce resources and valued knowledge of traditions, history and rites. When, thanks to modern healthcare and improvements in living standards, the number and proportion of older people in population increased, older people came under increased pressure to retire from active roles in society. Economic changes created new occupations which led to the loss of jobs, income and status by the aged. Urbanization contributed to the breakdown of the extended family, also leading to weaker family ties and lessening respect for older family members. The rise of mass education and literacy meant that there is no reverence for the aged on account of their superiority of knowledge. However, these changes could be interpreted as growing egalitarianism and individualism rather than as declining respect for older people, and it is highly questionable whether older people's status in all societies was in fact as high as the modernization theory suggests.

According to the *structured dependency theory*, society is structured in ways that make older people dependent, but in ways that lead some older people to be considerably more dependent than others (Estes 1979; Walker 1980 and 1981; Townsend 1981; Phillipson 1982; Evans and Williamson 1984). Lack of opportunities to work, poor pensions and institutional care make older people powerless and dependent. Poverty and female gender can serve to exacerbate this powerlessness and dependency. A possible criticism of the cruder versions of structured dependency theory is that it tends to present older people as powerless victims.

The *political economy of ageing* approach has many commonalities with the structured dependency theory as it stresses the ways in which political, economic and in particular (social) policy structures serve to render older people weak and marginalized. For instance, the forced or perceived need to exit from work is portrayed as a major cause for older people's marginalization in society. Dependence of older people is in this perspective socially constructed by governments and markets ('capitalism') that have acted in ways that have marginalized, dominated and weakened older people. We will return to examine questions that are highly relevant for this perspective in Chapters 6 and 10, where a number of policy challenges are used to illustrate the key roles that governments play in influencing the experience of ageing at individual and societal levels.

It is perhaps an inevitable result of the diversity of older populations and the multiplicity of approaches that can be taken to studying them that viable, falsifiable and widely tested (and accepted) theories of ageing have not arisen. Indeed, it should perhaps be accepted that the starting point of studying people selected on the basis of their age alone may not constitute a viable basis for theory building. However, this should not be viewed as discouraging ageing research but rather as an incentive to investigate the ways in which age interacts with other factors to produce outcomes that clearly matter in people's lives and that are, at least to some extent, modifiable.

Conclusion

This chapter has highlighted the importance of approaching the phenomenon of ageing from a number of different perspectives. It is not sufficient to view ageing merely as a demographic phenomenon in isolation from the social, political and economic factors surrounding ageing populations. Population ageing has been caused by a complex set of factors, and ageing in turn continues to have a very powerful impact on virtually all aspects of our lives, whether we are young or old ourselves. Population ageing has an impact on the society, politics and the economy, and vice versa. It has been said that the twentieth century was the period during which childhood and children's position and rights in society came under radical review; many signs are pointing in the direction of the twenty-first century being the period during which ageing and older people will demand a fundamental reassessment of attitudes towards ageing and of the policy measures that governments take in response to ageing. The exact shape of this 'silver century' is uncertain as yet and the ramifications of ageing are only partially visible and understood today. This book is intended as an aid to those who wish to gain an overview of the societal aspects of ageing, a phenomenon that is arguably, together with other major developments such as global warming and international conflict resolution, one of the most significant challenges of our times. In contrast to these other important issues, however, ageing is fundamentally a positive fact: while it does call for changes in policies, practices and attitudes (in this way it is very similar to, for example, environmental issues), it should also be highlighted as being one of humankind's most positive and remarkable achievements.

2 Demography 101: why do populations age?

Introduction

Chapter 1 briefly sketched out the main features of the demographic transition that has led societies to age. This chapter explores in greater depth the main features of this transition that has resulted in ageing societies and illustrates these in the form of graphs and tables. The chapter emphasizes the fact that while ageing is a global phenomenon, the timing and speed of the demographic transition vary across countries and parts of the world. While this chapter is therefore mindful of the delayed and compressed ageing process in many developing countries, it will focus on ageing in developed countries where the ageing process has already reached a very advanced stage and where many long-standing policies are being reformed in response to population ageing. This chapter focuses on the basic facts and figures of ageing from the demographic perspective. Chapter 6 will introduce terms and definitions (such as 'the old age dependency ratio') that are commonly used to measure and illustrate the 'burden' of ageing, often for the purposes of trying to justify adjustments in public spending on the older population.

Why are populations ageing?

A child born today in most parts of the world can expect to live longer than his or her parents. Many older people alive today would not have reached such an old age in the past. Whereas centenarians were exceedingly rare even in the recent past, in 2000 there were an estimated 167,000 centenarians in the world and by 2050 they are projected to number 3.3 million. Why is this the case?

To simplify somewhat, population ageing is the result of a transition from high birth rates and high death rates to low(er) birth rates and low(er) death rates. (Population age structure can also be influenced by inward and outward migration and major man-made or natural disasters such as earthquakes and wars, but we will not discuss these here as they currently have secondary, and in most cases only rather marginal, impact on the process of population ageing.) This chapter presents a number of tables, graphs and explanations in order to illustrate these complex processes. We start by outlining the transition from high to low(er) mortality and the resultant longer life expectancies at both younger and older ages.

Drivers of population ageing I

Lower mortality

In the demographic transition, declines in mortality usually precede declines in fertility. In other words, once fewer people are perishing (at young ages), people start having fewer children (for a variety of reasons). This model is somewhat idealized; in many developing countries, the temporal gap between these declines has been very small and they have tended to overlap somewhat. Whereas in the past the bulk of the gains in life expectancy were achieved through lower mortality among children, more recently the gains (especially in the more developed countries) have been made at the other end of the age spectrum – by lengthening the lives of older adults. Demographers Oeppen and Vaupel (2002) have estimated that life expectancy in the 'oldest' countries (where people live longest) has increased with a surprisingly regular rate of 2.5 years per decade since 1840. Oeppen and Vaupel (2002: 1029) argue that the four-decade increase in life expectancy since 1840 'may be the most remarkable regularity of mass endeavour ever observed'. Although a large number of variables have contributed to this development, the most important factors driving the increase in life expectancy are better health in the womb (through better nutrition and healthcare during pregnancy), better early childhood health, improved lifestyles for some sections of the population (e.g., less smoking), fewer physically exhausting and hazardous jobs, better nutrition and hygiene, better education and better medical care.

The 'increasingly rectangular survival curve' (see Figure 2.1 below) illustrates the fact that an increasing proportion of child and adult populations are now surviving until old or even very old age thanks to improved nutrition, hygiene and healthcare. Whereas many of the babies that were born in the past did not survive beyond the first and second years of life due to illness and malnutrition, infant mortality has been brought down to very low levels in the developed world. It is hard to imagine in the present day developed world the utter misery of childhoods blighted by disease and death and (female) reproductive lives ended prematurely (in the mother's death) or characterized by frequent pregnancy related complications and nursing of babies who in many cases perished before they reached 1 year of age. Whereas many individuals in the developed world now reach a rather advanced age without any personal experience of death (for instance, all the grandparents, parents, siblings and children of a 35-year-old of may still be alive), death used to be a very frequent experience in the lives of most people until relatively recently, and the death of children in particular greatly added to the misery and arduousness of human existence. As a result of survival into old age having become the standard life experience, the clear majority of people now die in old age, and a significant proportion do so following only a short period of disease and disability. 'Morbidity compression' refers to the delayed onset of morbidity (disease) until the period shortly before death – where most people reach a very old age, and are sick or disabled only for a short period before death; we will discuss this in more detail in Chapter 6.

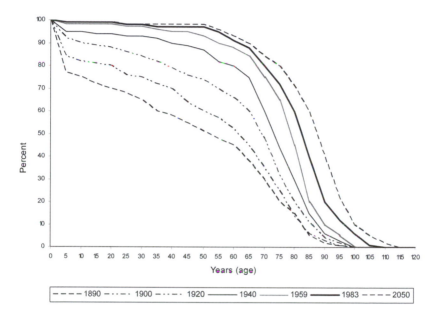

Source: Adapted from Laslett (1996: 60), fig. V.2.

Figure 2.1 The increasingly rectangular survival curve

Life expectancy

As a result of declines in mortality, life expectancies have increased. The term 'life expectancy' refers to the number of years that individuals in a particular population (typically that of a country or a region) or a population subgroup (typically based on gender and/or age) can expect to live, assuming that they adhere to the average pattern as based on past evidence and future projections of lifespans. While calculating the average across a large number of countries masks the considerable inter-country differences and can therefore be somewhat misleading, it is nonetheless striking to note that the average life expectancy across all the countries of the world has increased from 46.6 years in 1950–55 to 66.5 years in 2005–10 (United Nations 2007a).

Life expectancy can be estimated at different stages of an individual's or population cohort's life. *Life expectancy at birth* refers to the number of years that a newborn baby is estimated to live on average, provided that the age specific mortality rates prevailing at the time of the birth remain the same. However, it is increasingly important and interesting to have information about life expectancy not only among the newborns but also among older individuals. While the average life expectancy at birth in a given country may be, say, 72, individuals who have reached the age of 65 can on average expect to live considerably longer than for the seven years (72 minus 65) that would seem to remain on the basis of the average life expectancy at birth. This is because the life expectancy at birth figures take into account mortality in childhood and during earlier parts of adulthood: individuals who have survived to old age are obviously not affected by mortality at these earlier stages of life, and once they have 'made it this far', can expect to live longer on average than the population as a whole ('survivor effect'). The life expectancy of the 'oldest old' is even more at variance with life expectancy for the population as a whole: they tend to be members of a 'biological elite' that is often genetically predisposed and/or socially and economically favoured in ways that help them to enjoy a longer life than individuals who have died earlier. Chapter 4 will discuss the variance in (healthy) life expectancy by socioeconomic group in greater detail.

Drivers of population ageing II

Lower fertility

The other major driver of population ageing is the shift from high to low(er) fertility rates. Fertility rates have been declining for a long period in most developed countries and have now reached very low levels, in almost all cases below the 'replacement rate' of 2.1 children per woman. At the rate of 2.1, the population of 'reproductive age' is replacing itself by yielding two 'new' people per a woman and a 'corresponding' male, the 0.1 allowing for some mortality in childhood. Policymakers have for some time been grappling with the seemingly insurmountable challenge of reversing the trend towards lower fertility (this topic is further explored in Chapter 6 as we discuss the strategies that have been proposed to ameliorate population ageing). However, as Table 2.1 below indicates, falling fertility rates are not confined to the developed countries: the recent decades have witnessed a remarkable reduction of fertility levels in the less developed regions also, with total fertility falling from 5.41 to 2.75 children per woman. Fertility in the less developed regions is expected to reach replacement level (2.1 children on average per woman) around the middle of the twenty-first century and to fall below it thereafter. While fertility rates are clearly converging across the world, considerable differences in fertility rates are still expected to be in evidence in the middle of this century between the least developed countries (where comparatively high fertility rates are likely to be sustained) and the rest of the developing world where rates will be very similar to those in the developed world.

Table 2.1 Total fertility (children per woman) for the world, major areas and continents, 1970–75, 2005–10 and 2045–50 (medium forecast)

Major area	1970–75	2005–10	Medium forecast for 2045–50
World	4.47	2.55	2.0
More developed regions	2.13	1.60	1.8
Less developed regions	5.41	2.75	2.07
Africa	6.72	4.67	2.5
Asia	5.04	2.34	1.9
Europe	2.16	1.45	1.8
Latin America and the Caribbean	5.04	2.37	1.9
Northern America	2.01	2.00	1.9
Oceania	3.23	2.30	1.9

Source: Adapted from United Nations (2007a: 7), tab. 2, (2007b: 25), tab. II.1.

Table 2.1 obviously masks the diversity within the very large 'more developed' and 'less developed' regions and between countries within the continents. Table 2.2 below compares the average number of children per woman in 1970–75 with projections for the middle of the twenty-first century across a number of OECD and non-OECD countries. Current diversity notwithstanding, the most striking observation that can be made from this table is the dramatic convergence in predicted fertility rates *across* the OECD and non-OECD countries listed here to a level that is clearly below the replacement rate. The most common projection of 1.85 is obviously 'just' a projection, and therefore uncertain and as yet unproven, but past and present patterns point strongly in the direction of this being a reasonable estimate. While fertility rates have differed considerably in the past, it is reasonable to expect them to become strikingly similar for the large majority of the richer countries in the next 50 years or so.

Table 2.2   Total fertility (children per woman) in selected OECD and non-OECD countries

	1970–75	2045–50
OECD countries		
Australia	2.54	1.85
Austria	2.02	1.80
Belgium	1.93	1.75
Finland	1.62	1.85
France	2.31	1.85
Germany	1.64	1.74
Korea (Republic)	4.28	1.54
Mexico	6.60	1.85
Portugal	2.75	1.85
Turkey	5.30	1.85
United Kingdom	2.04	1.85
United States	2.02	1.85
Non-OECD countries		
China	4.86	1.85
India	5.43	1.85
Singapore	2.62	1.64
South Africa	5.47	1.85

Source: Adapted from United Nations (2007b: 73), tab. A.15.

Lower fertility + lower mortality = population ageing

As mortality rates have declined alongside declining birth rates, the share of older people in the population has increased in relation to the share of younger people. Indeed, a historic reversal in the proportions of 'the young' (those aged under 15) and 'the old' (those aged 60 and over) has taken place in the developed world, and is set to take place in the rest of the world by 2050. This increase in the proportion of the 60+ population persisted throughout the twentieth century worldwide, and this trend is set to continue into the foreseeable future.

As a result of lower birth rates and increased survival rates for older generations, the shape of the population structure in many countries has changed from a 'pyramid' to a 'pillar' (see Figure 2.2 below). In some cases, the lowest parts of the 'pillar' are narrower than the middle parts, reflecting strong declines in birth rates.

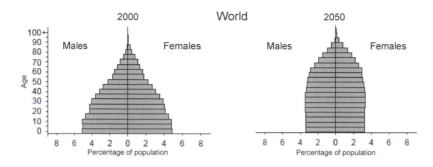

Figure 2.2 Population pyramids: age and sex distribution, 2000 and 2050

Source: United Nations (1999).

Pace of population ageing

Globally, the population of older persons is growing by approximately 2 percent every year, much faster than the population as a whole. For at least the next 25 years, the older population is expected to continue growing more rapidly than younger age groups. As can be seen from the figures in Box 2.1 below, the global number of individuals aged 60 or over tripled between 1950 and 2000, and is set to grow even faster during the next four–five decades, reaching two billion around the year 2050.

Box 2.1 Proportion of total population (%) and number (millions) of people aged 60 and over, worldwide, 1950–2050

1950	8%	200 million
2000	10%	600 million
2050	21%	2000 million

Source: Adapted from Mujahid (2006).

Older populations in the developing and developed countries

Demographic profiles and both the extent and speed of population ageing vary widely in different parts of the world: all share the general trend of ageing but are at different stages of the demographic transition and are progressing at different rates. Wilson (2000: 32) has identified the following five main patterns:

1   *Relatively slow ageing of an already aged population*: prime example of this is Western Europe that manifests slowly falling or static birth rates and slowly falling death rates.

2   *Intermediate rate of ageing: as above, plus possible reduction in traditionally high immigration*: examples of this pattern are the US, Australia and Canada.

3   *Very rapid ageing as a result of fast drop in birth rates and accelerating fall in death rates*: this pattern has been exemplified by Japan, parts of Latin America and China.

4   *Relatively slow ageing of a previously young population as a result of drop in birth rates and accelerating fall in death rates*: many developing countries and newly industrialized countries adhere to this pattern.

5   *Slow population ageing from an intermediate position as a result of low birth rates and static or even rising death rates*: former Soviet Union and parts of Eastern Europe developed this pattern as a result of a sudden and dramatic fall in (male) life expectancy following the fall of communism and the disintegration of social structures and health-care systems.

The fact that the absolute number of older people (defined as those aged 60 and over) in developing countries far outweighs the number of people in this age group in the developed world comes as a surprise to most people as we are used to thinking of the populations of poorer countries as 'young' and the populations of richer countries as 'old'. In fact, of the global population of approximately 600 million people aged 60 and over, some 400 million, or two-thirds, live in developing countries (an increase from approximately 50 percent in 1960). The *absolute* increase in the 60+ population will be less marked in the more developed regions, where the number of older persons is projected to rise from 232 million in 2000 to 394 million in 2050, but it will be dramatic in the less developed regions where the older population is predicted to more than quadruple, from 375 million in 2000 to 1.5 billion in 2050 (United Nations 2005). The pace of ageing is therefore considerably faster in developing countries than in developed countries. Many developing countries are also affected by the double burden of disease (co-existence of infectious and chronic diseases), and the lower level of economic development in developing countries makes it harder for them to offer ageing populations the assistance that they need. In view of this fact, the alarmist reaction to population ageing in many rich countries seems ill-placed and exaggerated, even hysterical: there can be no doubt that the real challenges lie in responding to the needs of the ageing populations of poor countries (see Oppong (2006) for a sobering description of the difficulties faced in Sub-Saharan Africa by older women in particular).

While the absolute number of older people in the developing world far outweighs the number of older people in the developed world, the percentage share of the total population constituted by older people is greater in developed countries. In the more developed regions of the world, approximately 20 percent of the population was aged 60 years or older in 2000. By 2050, this proportion is expected to have increased to one-third. In the less developed regions of the world, the proportion is expected increase from 8 percent to nearly 20 percent between 2000 and 2050. Table 2.3 illustrates the fact that while the proportions of the total populations constituted by people aged 60 and over are converging, the differences are likely to remain large. For example, the share of the 60+ population is predicted to exceed 40 percent in Japan and Korea, but is forecast to reach a much lower proportion in some other developed countries such as Australia, Denmark and the United States (this is largely due to higher birth rates and stronger net migration that boost the share of the younger populations in these countries). Growth in the share of the older population will be most remarkable in countries that at present have relatively low proportions of their population in the 60+ category: in Korea and Mexico the predicted proportion is almost 20 percentage points higher than the current share of the 60+ population. While the share of the older population is predicted to grow in African countries also, this share is believed to reach a comparatively very low level: in South Africa, one of the continent's richest countries, it is predicted to be as low as 14 percent.

Table 2.3 Percentage distribution of the population in selected age groups, by country, age group 60+, 2005 and 2050 (medium variant)

	Age group 60+ (%), 2005	Age group 60+ (%), 2050
OECD countries		
Australia	17.8	30.2
Austria	21.9	35.3
Czech Republic	19.9	38.6
Denmark	21.2	29.4
Germany	25.1	37.0
Greece	23.3	38.1
Hungary	20.8	34.4
Italy	25.3	38.6
Japan	26.4	44.0
Korea	13.7	42.2
Mexico	8.4	27.3
Poland	17.2	39.6
Slovakia	16.1	37.6
Spain	21.7	39.0
Turkey	8.2	24.5
United States	16.6	26.8

Non-OECD countries		
China	11.0	31.1
India	7.5	20.2
Singapore	12.3	39.8
South Africa	6.7	13.8

Source: Adapted from United Nations (2007b: 60–4), tab. A.10.

Growing and shrinking populations

The world population is expected to increase by 2.6 billion during the next 44 years, from 6.5 billion today to 9.1 billion in 2050. The world population is growing by 1.2 percent annually, implying a net addition of 77 million people per year. Whereas today the population of the more developed regions of the world is rising at an annual rate of 0.30 percent, that of the less developed regions is increasing nearly five times as fast, at 1.4 percent, and the subset of the 49 least developed countries is experiencing even more rapid growth (2.4 percent per year, with a still robust annual rate of 1.3 percent predicted for 2045–50).

While world population is therefore set to increase fast over the next 50 years, the populations of some countries will in fact decline. In contrast to the predicted increase in the world population, the population of the 27 countries that were EU members in 2007 is predicted to fall by 7 percent to approximately 454 million by the middle of the twenty-first century. Population decline is expected to be dramatic in countries with particularly low fertility (despite significant net migration in some cases). Because fertility levels for most of the developed countries are expected to remain below the replacement level in 2000–50, the populations of 30 developed countries are projected to be smaller by mid-century than today: 14 percent smaller in Japan, 22 percent smaller in Italy, and 30–50 percent smaller in Bulgaria, Estonia, Latvia, the Russian Federation and Ukraine. The Deutsche Bank of Germany (2002) has predicted that even assuming annual immigration of 250,000 people, the German population will decline to 50 million by 2100 (it is currently 80 million). The possible and actual responses to these developments and their implications are further discussed in Chapter 6.

Median age

In addition to the percentage of the older population in the total population, the extent and pace of population ageing can be gauged via the median age. The term 'median' refers to the middle number in a sequence of numbers. The median age in a population cuts the population in half: half of the population are younger than the persons of median age and the other half are older.

Upward or downward shifts in the median age are therefore a good indicator of the progression of population ageing. The median age in the world today is 28. According to United Nations projections for 2050, the world median age will be 38. At present, the youngest country in the world is Yemen with a median age of 15. Japan, with a median age of 42.9, is currently the country with the oldest population in the world, followed by Italy, Switzerland, Germany and Sweden with median ages of about 40 years each. In 2050, Japan is projected to maintain its title as having the oldest population, with a median age of 54.9 years. Armenia, the Czech Republic, Estonia, Greece, Italy, Latvia, Singapore, Slovenia and Spain, with median ages greater than 51 years in 2050 will also have populations where persons aged 50 or over predominate.

Table 2.4 Median age by major area, 1950, 2000, 2050

	1950	2005	2050
World total	23.9	28.0	38.1
More developed regions	29.0	38.6	45.7
Less developed regions	21.5	25.5	36.9
Least developed countries	19.5	19.0	27.9
Africa	19.1	19.0	28.0
Asia	22.2	27.6	40.2
Latin America and Caribbean	20.0	26.0	40.1
Europe	29.7	38.9	47.3
North America	29.8	36.3	41.5
Oceania	28.0	32.3	40.0

Source: United Nations (2007b), tab. I.4.

Table 2.5 Median age by country, 1950, 2005, 2050

	Median age, 1950	Median age, 2005	Median age, 2050
OECD countries			
World	23.9	28.0	38.1
Canada	27.7	38.6	45.3
Finland	27.7	40.9	44.4
France	34.5	38.9	44.7
Hungary	29.9	38.7	48.1
Ireland	29.6	33.4	43.0
Italy	29.0	42.0	50.4
Japan	22.3	42.9	54.9
Korea	19.1	35.0	54.9
Slovakia	27.3	35.6	51.0
United Kingdom	34.6	38.9	43.4

Non-OECD countries

China	23.9	32.5	45.0
India	21.3	23.8	38.6
Singapore	20.0	37.5	53.7
South Africa	20.9	23.9	30.2

Source: Adapted from United Nations (2007b: 66–70), tab. A.12.

The ageing of the aged

The older population itself is ageing. The fastest growing age group in the world is the 'oldest old' (individuals aged 80 years and over) who currently constitute one-tenth of the total number of older persons in the world. By 2050, the share of the oldest old of the global older population (i.e., the share of people aged 80 or over of the population aged 65 or over) is expected to be one-fifth.

In 2000, 69 million persons in the world were aged 80 or over, and they were the fastest growing segment of population. By 2050 they are projected to reach 377 million, increasing more than 5.5 times from the 2000 level. Although the proportion of the oldest old is still low as a percentage share (1.1 percent of world population), it is projected to rise to 4.2 percent in 2050. In Sweden, 5.1 percent of the population is already aged 80 or over, while in Denmark, Norway, Switzerland and the UK their share is over 4 percent.

In 2050, 21 countries or areas are projected to have at least 10 percent of their population aged 80 years or over (octogenarians, nonagenarians and centenarians): these countries include, among others, Austria, Belgium, Cuba, Finland, France, Germany, Greece, Hong Kong SAR of China, Italy, Japan, the Republic of Korea, Singapore, Slovenia, Spain, Sweden and Switzerland. Five countries are predicted to have more than ten million people aged 80 and over: China (98 million), India (47 million), US (29 million), Japan (17 million) and Brazil (13 million) (United Nations 2002).

Large numbers of people reaching the milestone of 100 years is a very novel phenomenon. In 2000 there were an estimated 167,000 centenarians in the world; by 2050 they are projected to number 3.3 million. Japan will have the highest proportion of centenarians in 2050 (nearly 1 percent of its population). It will be followed by France, Norway, Sweden and Switzerland. In 2050 the largest centenarian populations are predicted to be found in Japan (1,016,000), the US (471,000), China (459,000), India (131,000), France (123,000) and Germany (114,000). Given the size of the market, it is fair to assume that birthday card stands in the stationery shops of many countries will soon start carrying a range of 100th birthday cards!

Table 2.6 Percentage distribution of the population in selected age groups, by country, age group 80+, 2005 and 2050 (medium variant)

	Age group 80+ (%), 2005	Age group 80+ (%), 2050
OECD countries		
Australia	3.5	9.3
Austria	4.3	11.9
Belgium	4.3	10.7
Canada	3.5	10.0
Czech Republic	3.1	9.0
Denmark	4.1	9.2
Finland	4.0	10.0
France	4.6	10.2
Germany	4.4	13.1
Greece	3.5	11.4
Hungary	3.2	7.2
Iceland	3.0	9.6
Ireland	2.7	6.7
Italy	5.1	13.3
Japan	4.8	15.5
Korea	1.4	12.7
Mexico	1.2	6.0
Netherlands	3.6	10.4
New Zealand	3.2	9.2
Norway	4.6	9.0
Poland	2.7	8.9
Portugal	3.7	10.1
Slovakia	2.4	7.9
Spain	4.3	12.2
Sweden	5.3	9.3
Switzerland	4.3	11.0
Turkey	0.6	3.8
United Kingdom	4.5	9.2
United States	3.5	7.6
Non-OECD countries		
China	1.2	7.3
India	0.7	3.1
Singapore	1.5	14.8
South Africa	0.5	2.2

Source: Adapted from United Nations (2007b: 60–4), tab. A.10.

Gender balance among the aged

In the past, the gender balance in older age groups used to be roughly equal. As a result of declining maternal mortality (i.e., death during pregnancy, in childbirth or in the postnatal period) and other factors (including a possibly greater genetic disposition to longer lives and exogenous factors such as healthier lifestyles among women), a gap in life expectancies in favour of women emerged and widened in the twentieth century in many countries. As a result of this difference in life expectancies, the majority of older persons are women, and the gender imbalance grows with age. In 2000 there were 63 million more women than men in the world aged 60 or older. As Box 2.2 below indicates, this female majority increases with age so that only some 18 percent of centenarians are men. Given that the majority of these women in the oldest age groups are in most countries widowed and often also living alone, the question of organizing care and support for them becomes very important – we will return to this issue in Chapters 3, 7 and 8 that analyse inter-generational relations and long term care respectively.

Box 2.2   Proportion of women among different age groups, worldwide, 2007

49–50	50%
60+	55%
80+	64%
100+	82%

Source: Adapted from United Nations (2007c), fig. III.

Conclusion

Population ageing results from the demographic transition, which is a phenomenon that virtually all countries in the world have come to share, albeit at different times, at varying speeds and with some differences in the sequence of shifts in birth and death rates. The previous situation where higher birth rates and higher death rates prevailed resulted in pyramid shaped population structures, whereas the population structures in many countries are now beginning to look more like pillars, or even something approximating an inverted pyramid. Death rates are still falling in virtually all countries in the world. There is more variation in the rate at which birth rates are falling. The transition to low birth rates took place earlier in Europe than in most other places in the world, but also took longer. In Japan, for instance, the transition from relatively high to very low birth rates took place in one generation. In France, this process took more than a century. Developing countries face particular challenges when adjusting to ageing populations as not only is the speed of demographic transition faster than it was in societies that aged earlier, but the infrastructure of services and benefits needed to support ageing populations is in many cases lacking or inadequate. In the developed countries where such an infrastructure of services and benefits for older people was put in place and expanded during the twentieth century, the challenge is perceived differently, namely in terms of adjusting that infrastructure in a manner that makes ageing more 'affordable'. Chapters 5 and 6 will discuss the validity of the argument that population ageing necessitates radical welfare state retrenchment and will also review the various policy options that governments have at their disposal when responding to population ageing. However, as this chapter has pointed out, it is clear that the greatest challenges in the area of population ageing are to be found in the world's poorest countries where *expansion* of support for older people is desperately needed: the 'problems' associated with ageing societies in the rich world are clearly miniscule in comparison.

3   Changing family structures and inter-generational solidarity

Introduction

This chapter discusses the evolving social and family contexts of ageing. It stands to reason that the extent to which an older person is enmeshed in a social network has a strong influence on his or her experience of ageing. While the 'social' context of ageing obviously extends beyond families into friends, neighbours and the full range of social activities that people undertake, we cannot gain a full understanding of ageing in a social context without knowledge of trends and developments in the structure of families. Here, again, there is a strong connection between 'older' and 'younger' individuals in that there tends to be extensive channeling of both financial and non-financial supports between the members of different generations in a family (including transfers from the older to the younger generations that are often overlooked). Family structures have a fundamental impact on the support and help networks available to older people, and changes therein will lead to changes in the experience of old age in the future. Patterns of marriage and divorce, the increasing prevalence of living alone, and the declining level of fertility have an impact on the social networks and support structures of older people today and in the decades to come. However, the chapter cautions against adopting a naive view of the past and a gloomy view of the future: while social isolation and loneliness do affect some older people in modern societies, there is no reason to believe that developments such as smaller family size or even increased prevalence of divorce will necessarily result in more pronounced social isolation among the older populations in the future. Personal communities – friends and acquaintances who are not family members but act as central sources of support – play a significant role for some groups of older people (especially the urban and middle-class older people – Phillipson et al. 2001), and this trend may become stronger in the future. For instance, childless individuals may develop strong patterns of establishing and cultivating 'families of choice' that they associate with and draw support from throughout the lifecourse.

From the bosom of the extended family to loneliness and social exclusion?

Many people hold a comfortable image that in the past societies were characterized by extended families where the old, those in middle years and the young shared households and made their different contributions to the smooth functioning of the three generational living arrangements, lovingly looking after all who needed care. This image is then frequently contrasted with the modern day scenario of lonely older people neglected by their families who are too busy working and devoting themselves to leisure activities. The idealized view of the past as a time when living in the midst of an extended family ensured a happy and secure old age is both highly simplistic and largely false (see, e.g., Thane 1998, 2000). No single type of household or family type typified the pre-industrial society. Laslett (1996) has argued that the three generation household was a comparative rarity in most pre-industrial societies (although it appears to have been more common for instance in Asia than in Europe). One of the obvious reasons for this comparative rarity of *three* generation households is that, due to shorter life expectancies, many people did not survive to see their grandchildren.

In most parts of the world old age spent in three generational families has therefore been a considerably rarer phenomenon than is often thought. However, two generational (ageing parent with adult child(ren)) households used to be more common: until recently a large proportion of older people used to co-reside with surviving children, and still do so in many countries. According to Costa (1998), in 1880 in America approximately half of retired men lived with their children; by 1990 this proportion had dropped to 5 percent. Studies of older people's lives in the United Kingdom in the 1940s and 1950s also show that co-residence between two or (less commonly) three generations used to be fairly prevalent (although the shortage of housing in the post-Second World War period and the relatively deprived nature of the areas studied obviously influenced the prevalence of co-residence in these studies): Sheldon (1948) reported in his study of Wolverhampton that half of the older people lived in two or three generation households; Townsend's (1957) study of Bethnal Green in London estimated this proportion as 40 percent. An important part of the explanation for this is the fact that child-bearing often went on until an older age than at present, and many older people were living with their adult children because some of them had not yet left home to marry and establish their own households (for instance a woman who had a child at the age of 45 might still live with that child when she reached the age of 65). Also, poverty often prevented older people from running their own households, particularly after the death of the (working) spouse. Poverty and lack of alternatives to co-residence are still important contributing factors to extensive co-residence between ageing parents and adult children in the developing countries: where the incomes of older people are improved (as they were following a pensions reform in Brazil in the 1990s), older people display a pattern of choosing to establish their own separate households (Kamiya 2006).

Household structures: living alone or in a single generation household

Living arrangements have in many countries evolved so that two generation and three generation households have become considerably rarer than in the past. Residence in multigenerational households has been largely replaced by households consisting of older couples or single person households. However, living arrangements differ greatly between countries. For instance, in Korea and Singapore three generational households are still the most common household type for older persons, and in China co-residence with an adult son (and his family) is widespread. Even in the 'Western' countries there are striking differences between countries in the prevalence of co-residence and single person households. The current situation where a very large proportion of the older population of many developed countries live for very long periods of time on their own or with their spouse is a historically novel phenomenon, brought about by increased wealth, increased life expectancy and changed preferences.

There are several reasons for the growing numbers of older people who live alone or in households consisting of older people only (most typically a married couple). Living alone is more common among older women than among older men because they tend to live longer, and are therefore in many instances 'left behind' by their deceased spouses and partners. For instance, whereas approximately three-quarters of older men in the UK are married, half of older women are widowed. These patterns clearly have significant implications for patterns of residence as well as informal care in view of the fact that spouses are becoming an increasingly important source of care.

It is important to appreciate that, in most cases, older people living alone are in this household form voluntarily. Living alone is usually a choice, rather than an imposition, and does not in itself imply isolation or vulnerability. Indeed, some older people have always lived alone; many others find the alternatives to living alone highly unpalatable. The introduction of modern pension schemes lessened the need to form multigenerational households by giving older people a greater degree of economic independence than in the past. However, the most important reason for the proliferation of households consisting of older persons is the preference of most older people in developed countries for independent living rather than extended family living arrangements: shared living between adult children and older parents is not considered desirable (or necessary) by most people. Survey evidence indicates that older people like to see their children regularly and to live nearby, but not to share a house with them. 'Intimacy at a distance' is a phrase coined by the sociologists Rosenmayr (1977) to describe this preference for independent living arrangements with access to support and social interaction where necessary and desirable.

Arguably more important than co-residence is the geographical distance between adult children and ageing parents, and in particular the frequency of contact between them (which is partly influenced, but not exclusively determined, by distance). In some contexts, mobility trends point in the direction of a greater dispersion of kin. As Table 3.1 below indicates, there are considerable differences between European countries in the degree to which older people are geographically removed from their children. Whereas co-residence is still fairly common in Italy (and other Mediterranean countries), it has become exceedingly rare in Sweden (and other Nordic countries). However, total family dispersion is very unusual, and dispersion beyond one and a half hours' travel time is not characteristic of the large majority of older people's immediate families in most countries and areas. Severe dispersion is a far from typical experience and is not on a sharp rise. Furthermore, while distance between parents and children does matter when it comes to care giving, it is not the only relevant factor: the children's employment status and the presence of children also matter (Wolf et al. 1997).

Table 3.1 indicates that while daily contact between older adults and their children tends to be more frequent in Italy (this is obviously in large part the result of co-residence), the proportion of older people who are in weekly or more frequent contact is in fact strikingly similar between these countries (Italy still has a lead, but not a very considerable one). Similarly, when the proportion of those who receive at least one type of help from their children or co-reside with children is calculated, the context of ageing in these disparate countries is surprisingly similar (France lags slightly behind but again the difference is not striking). In other words, differences in co-residence seem to mask very similar levels of interaction and assistance between the parental generation and adult children across Europe.

Table 3.1 Relationships between the 1945–54 cohort respondents and their ascendants

	Sweden	**Germany**	**France**	**Italy**
Proximity				
In same household	2.0	13.0	7.5	24.3
Less than 5 km	28.8	36.5	23.0	33.7
More than 5 km	69.2	50.5	69.5	41.9

Frequency of contact				
Daily	18.3	27.5	20.5	54.5
At least once a week	60.0	50.8	53.5	33.1
Less often	21.6	21.3	25.9	12.4
*Type of support**				
Personal care	6.7	8.3	5.5	12.9
Household help	34.2	28.8	18.5	14.3
At least one type of help	40.9	37.4	26.6	28.8
At least one type of help OR living in same household/building	42.0	41.5	32.0	42.3

Note: *Care given to persons outside household in previous 12 months.
Source: Adapted from Ogg and Renaut (2006).

We will now turn to examining some aspects of families and reproductive behaviour that are relevant from the point of view of older people's social networks, quality of life and social support.

Family and social changes that shape the experience of old age

Marriage and divorce: lonely old age?

Patterns of marriage and divorce influence the number of people who are seen to be 'alone' (although not necessarily childless, friendless or even partnerless) in old age. However, a number of factors need to be taken into account in order to obtain an accurate picture of the impact of marriage and divorce rates. In many societies co-habitation without marriage has become a popular choice that can persist into old age. For this reason, marriage statistics increasingly need to be accompanied by information about the proportion of people living in consensual unions or co-habiting. Divorce rates are not a particularly reliable guide to the future numbers of older people living without a spouse or a partner. If divorce is followed by remarriage, the result may not be just the presence of a partner in old age but also the presence of a new kind of 'extended' or 'reconstituted' family with children (and other relatives) from the previous unions and possibly the new union also. Note also that the prevalence of this kind of 'reconstituted families' may not increase overall: whereas previously family reconstitution followed the death of a spouse, reconstituted families are now increasingly commonly the result of remarriage or repartnering following divorce or separation (although it has to be admitted that the 'issues' that can arise in the union following the former spouse's death are quite different from those that arise in a postdivorce or postseparation scenario where the former spouse is still alive, and possibly establishing a new family unit which may or may not link in with the old one).

Given that 'reconstituted families' formed as a result of divorce and remarriage are a relatively new phenomenon, it is too early to predict what their impact on life in older age is. However, it is probably safe to say that the potential expansion in the number of relationships in 'reconstituted families' does not automatically translate into increased support for older people. Whereas 'combining' children from previous and new relationships or marriages results in a larger total number is children that one is 'related to', this does not necessarily translate into the kind of ties of mutual obligation and affection that last until the (step)parent's old age (Dimmock et al. 2004). Similarly, it would be wrong to assume that divorce and remarriage dilute all feelings of affection, resulting in lack of support or contact with one's own children in old age. Indeed, there appear to be significant gender differences here. While divorce frequently leaves the relationship between the mother and child(ren) intact or even stronger than before, divorced fathers' contact with their children is often decimated, with negative consequences for contact, support and care in later life.

We do not know enough about postdivorce or postseparation relationships among older people as yet. While a large proportion of divorced and separated individuals form new marriages and partnerships, the proportion of those who remain alone appears to be increasing. Co-habitation of older adults may have a more stable and lasting nature than co-habitation among younger adults, and indeed many older adults may have a preference for a living apart together (LAT) relationship where a couple relationship is forged while the partners continue to live in their own homes (Borell and Ghazan-fareeon Karlsson).

The impact of increased divorce rates can of course extend beyond the child–parent relationship and is often seen as having a negative impact on the grandparent–grandchild relationship. Maintaining contact with grandchildren can become problematic following the parents' divorce or separation if the children remain with the former son- or daughter-in-law. Paternal grandparents, in particular, are at a greater risk of losing contact with their grandchildren following divorce or separation (largely for the simple reason that, postdivorce, children typically remain with their mother). However, it is also possible that divorce leads to a much closer relationship between a grandchild and (one or more of the) grandparents if some or even the bulk of the responsibility for raising the child is transferred to the grandparent(s) (Cox 2000). Similarly, the ageing parents of never married single parents can end up playing a central role in raising their grandchildren in the absence of the other parent.

Lower fertility rates: no children to turn to in old age?

As was pointed out in Chapter 2, the drop in fertility rates is one of the two important global trends that have brought about population ageing. It is tempting to think that this fall in the average number of children and the rise in childlessness will lead to old age being a lonely experience for many. But does the transition from high to low birth rates translate into lack of supports in old age?

It cannot be denied that childlessness or the absence of children in older age as a result of migration, divorce, family enmity, social mobility or the demands of family and work on the younger generations can constitute a painful experience for some older people (Kreager and Schroeder-Butterfill 2005). However, several factors will mitigate the impact of smaller family size on the availability of support in old age. First it is important to bear in mind that of the larger number of children born to previous generations, fewer survived to the age where they could be useful to their parents in old age. Also, while it may be the case that the amount of support received from children in old age is positively related to the number of children, the marginal benefits from each additional child beyond the second or the third child are in most cases very small. Rather, the critical distinction is between having none versus some children, and second between having one versus having two or more children. Where there are few children in a family, more may be required of each child, but the relationships between children and parents may also be closer than in large families. In other words, when studying changing family size we should pay less attention to changes in the mean number of children, and more attention to the proportion of people with no children or only one child (Uhlenberg 1993, 1995).

Data from the United States indicates that among women aged 85 and older, 25 percent have no children. The new cohorts entering old age in the next decades will in fact have a *smaller* proportion of childless people (although the share of the childless appears set to increase again when the cohorts that are currently nearing the end of their reproductive lives in many low fertility countries enter old age). Current levels of childlessness are not historically unprecedented: whereas for previous generations the primary reasons for childlessness in old age were poverty or high infant (and adult) mortality, the primary reason currently lies in individual and lifestyle choices, in other words, the deliberate decision to remain childless. At an earlier stage in history, a woman may have given birth to, say, six children, but half of them may have died in infancy and the remaining three of diseases, in wars, accidents, and so on, before their mother reached old age (*if* the mother reached old age, that is). Furthermore, fertility rates are difficult to predict in the long term and fluctuation is possible. The proportion of people with no children or only one child is therefore prone to change: childlessness may decline among the next generation, only to increase again.

From adult children to spouse carers

It is important to note that the decline in the average number of children is in many countries compensated for by the greater propensity of older people to be married and by greater longevity among both men and women: whereas in the past a widowed mother may have needed to turn to her child(ren) for support and assistance, spouses are now becoming an increasingly important source of family care in old age. Furthermore, the childless adult children, unencumbered by responsibilities towards a younger generation, may also become one of the 'new' sources of help and support to their ageing parents. The alarm about shrinking numbers of children leading to a care deficit is therefore overstated.

Peter Townsend (1957) describes in his seminal book on the family and community lives of old people in Bethnal Green, London, the co-existence and in many case the co-residence of two or even three generations in a working class urban environment in the 1950s. A repeat study of older persons' lives in the same area carried out 50 years later found that the 'companionate marriage' had become the central focus of most older persons' lives and that two or three generation households had become very rare. This finding reflects the shift in the sources of support from adult children (and the daughter–mother relationship in particular) to spouses. This, of course, means that often those who provide care and support to older people are older themselves, and may therefore require support in their caring role. Another development that has led to an increase in the number of 'spouse carers' is the decline, in many countries, in the number of widows and the increase in the number of older women with partners (as a result of the narrowing gap in male and female life expectancies) (Pickard et al. 2000).

Overlapping generations: the beanpole family

The assumed disadvantages of family change for older generations are so entrenched in most people's thinking that they tend to gloss over the extension in the scope for inter-generational relationships. Increased longevity in combination with lower fertility has led to the verticalization of family structures (Harper 2004). This term denotes the longer and narrower family structures or what is sometimes called the 'beanpole family' in reference to the (longer) co-existence of (fewer members of) several generations. The likelihood that people in older age groups still have a surviving parent has increased: it has become the majority pattern to have a surviving parent at age 50 and it is increasingly common to have one even at the age of 60. Approximately one-quarter of 55–63-year-old British women have a surviving parent; in the United States this proportion of middle-aged women with a surviving parent is as high as 40 percent (Grundy 1999). Young adults, too, are more likely to have a grandparent who is still alive. In the United States, as many as half of the people aged 55 and over belong to four (or even five) generation families – they have a surviving parent, children and (great)-grandchildren (Bengtson et al. 1995). In the UK, three-quarters of individuals aged 60 or over belong to families with three or more generations (Grundy et al. 1999). However, the incidence of four to five generation families naturally depends on the age at which people have children – if the age of childbearing is around 35, it is highly unlikely that more than three generations will co-exist for any length of time. Very few individuals are currently members of five generation families and any increase in the prevalence of these particularly lengthy 'beanpoles' is dependent on a co-incidence of increased life expectancies and relatively young ages of (first) reproduction.

The duration of the period that people co-exist with members of different generations in their family has therefore been considerably extended. Many more individuals now stand a chance of building a long term relationship with their (great)grandchildren and (great)grandparents than was possible in the past. While the number of grandchildren is now smaller than in the past, more individuals survive to experience grandparenthood and many who do so have the opportunity to actually get to know their grandchildren/grandparents over long periods of time, in many cases amounting to several decades. Many individuals in the developed world now are in the role of a grandparent for a quarter of a century or even longer: this constitutes a great opportunity, in principle, for communication, learning and understanding between generations. The extensive contact between grandparents and grandchildren is illustrated by the finding that, in the UK, half of 50–9-year-olds with grandchildren see them weekly (although contact tends to diminish with advancing age as grandchildren grow older and less family centred in their activities) (Grundy et al. 1999).

The 'sandwich generation' and women's labour market participation

As was pointed out above, while people who reproduce have on average considerably fewer children than in the past, the likelihood of those children surviving until their parents' old age is now much greater, thanks to decreased death rates. Once the other parent has died, adult children in their late middle age tend to assume greater care responsibilities so that around the age of 55, many have a parent who needs some help and support (although the extent and nature of this support can vary considerably). However, contrary to a popular image, middle age is not a period of fulfilling constant and excessive demands for care by ageing parents. Drawing on data from the Health and Retirement Study in the United States, Johnson and Lo Sasso established that fewer than half of 53–63-year-old women had living parents and of these no more than 10 percent provided help to their parents amounting to more than 100 hours per year (Johnson and Lo Sasso 2004). In a Canadian study, across five-year age categories between the ages of 35 to 64, between 11–22 percent of daughters and 7–12 percent of sons provided at least one kind of help to their parents once a month or more often (the types of help were housework, transport, personal care, financial support, outside work/household maintenance). However, the need for personal care (washing, dressing, etc.) is clearly the most demanding type of care work and is the best indicator of a high degree of dependency. In the Canadian study, around 2 percent of 35–49-year-old daughters provided personal care to parents, the percentage rising to 5.6 percent for 50–54-year-old daughters (Gee and Gutman 2000).

It appears therefore to be the case that fairly significant proportions of middle aged individuals (and women in particular) are engaged in providing care services to their parents. The term 'sandwich generation' refers to a group of people who have care responsibilities towards both their own children and towards their parents. There is much debate and anecdotal evidence regarding this generation (also sometimes referred to as 'women in the middle'). The concept of a 'sandwich generation' also gives rise to a number of issues regarding the definition of being 'sandwiched'. What age of a child or how many children does a 'sandwiched' person have to have? Clearly, looking after a 2-year-old is rather different from looking after a 16-year-old, even if the latter still lives at home, and having five children is more demanding than having one. Do we also make holding a paid job outside the home a requirement for being sandwiched, and do we assume that adults engaged in home duties are better able to handle the pressures of being sandwiched?

In Canada (Gee and Gutman 2000), among daughters who had a parent alive *and* a child at home, the highest percentage in any age group who helped a parent at least once a month was 13 percent. In the potentially most problematic group – those who had a living parent, a child at home *and* a paid job – the highest percentage in any age group that helped a parent at least monthly was 7 percent. In other words, while the 'sandwiched' people clearly constitute a minority, there are significant numbers of people with multiple care and other commitments. It is particularly striking that in the light of some comparative statistics, the informal care inputs by people in paid employment do not differ significantly from informal care inputs by people outside paid employment.

Combining paid work and family responsibilities has become more common than in the past. The alleged crisis stemming from decreased supply of informal care givers as a result of women's increased employment outside the home is sometimes referred to as the 'care giving crunch'. However, as was pointed out above, there are minimal differences between employed and non-employed women in the type of help provided to parents and in the amount of time spent helping parents. This seems to indicate that care is still available despite changes in women's labour market participation rates, but it may be coming at a high cost to some individuals whose situation should be alleviated by policies designed to make the combination of care and work easier and more financially, physically and psychologically manageable (Phillips et al. 2002; see also Chapter 7). Receiving financial help from parents prior to care needs arising does increase the likelihood of providing care to the parents (Henretta et al. 1997). However, it would be grossly simplistic to view most care arrangements as 'payment' for money, support or services rendered in the past.

Older people's contributions to the resources and well being of younger relatives

Most data and debates focus on care and support given by younger people to older people – a prime example of how research and policy embody ageism (see also Chapter 9). However, it is important not to view social relations between families and older people as a one way process where older people are in need of and receive (or even demand, at whatever cost to others) various supports and services from younger relatives. Although they are rarely quantified, older people make very considerable care and financial inputs into their children's and grandchildren's lives, see, for instance, Hoff 2007. Research has shown that *financial* transfers within families are overwhelmingly from the older to the younger generation (Sundstrom et al. 1996). Even prior to death, in some countries (e.g., Ireland, Italy) it is not uncommon for parents to make very substantial contributions to their adult children's purchase of a first home and other major investments such as higher education (indeed it is sometimes argued that expectations of such extensive financial gifts to children have the effect of reducing fertility – only one child may be perceived to be 'affordable'). In the area of care, too, the emphasis is usually on care given by younger to older generations: this tends to divert attention away from the very extensive inputs that older generations have into the care of younger generations. The Health and Retirement Study (HRS) in the United States has established that parent to child transfers tend to peak around the age of 60, and that child to parent transfers become predominant from the age of 75 (Johnson and Lo Sasso 2004). We still know too little about the nature and quantity of these parent to child transfers of practical help and support and financial assistance.

Most contributions of older adults are therefore not systematically recorded. For this reason, they tend to go unnoticed and are usually taken for granted despite the fact that their role in underpinning the formal economy and economic development is crucial. One major area of 'downward' intergenerational transfers of time is 'grandparenting'. This covers a large and varied area of care giving that is often of crucial importance for working, lone or otherwise pressurized parents. As was pointed out above, divorce or lone parenthood in the adult child generation may increase the need for support from older parents. In many developing countries, extensive support is given by the older generation in the form of tangible household and childcare assistance (e.g., Hermalin et al. 1998; Schroeder-Butterfill 2003). In contemporary China, the fact that many working parents from rural areas have trusted virtually all childcare work to their ageing parents means that these grandparents are in a very real sense enabling and underpinning the current economic boom in China (Silverstein et al. 2006). In countries where the 'middle' generation is wiped out or incapacitated by HIV/AIDS, grandparents assume enormous responsibility for raising their grandchildren. Worldwide millions of children have been orphaned or made vulnerable by HIV/AIDS. The most affected region is Sub-Saharan Africa, where some 12.3 million children under the age of 18 have lost one or both parents by AIDS. A large share of these orphaned children is already living with their grandparents or other older care givers. For instance, in Namibia, the share of orphans (not living with a surviving parent) being taken care of by grandparents rose from 44 percent in 1992 to 61 percent in 2000. A similar pattern is in evidence in other countries such as Tanzania and Zimbabwe (UNAIDS, UNICEF and USAID 2004).

Inter-generational solidarity

It is often assumed that the younger generations are too absorbed in their busy lives to want any intensive involvement in the care of their parents. Older people are sometimes portrayed as being reluctant to pay themselves for the expensive medical and social care that they may need. Do research findings bear these assumptions out?

EU citizens' responses to survey questions regarding the best care arrangements for their own parents revealed significant differences between countries. Among the EU-15 member states, Ireland together with the Mediterranean member states had the lowest levels of support for formal care solutions for the respondents' own parents (including both formal home care and residential care). In contrast, the majority of respondents advocated a formal care solution for their own parents in (in descending order) Sweden, Denmark, the Netherlands, Finland, France and Belgium (Alber and Köhler 2004). The country specific availability and quality of formal services are most likely a powerful influence on these attitudes (see Chapter 7 for an elaboration of this argument on the impact of policy structures on preferences for and acceptability of different care alternatives).

While the difference between women's and men's preferences for increased family responsibility is rather slight, the differences between generations are clearer. Throughout the EU, older people are more in favour of

Table 3.2 Percentage of respondents advocating different care solutions for their own parents, selected EU countries

	Move together	**Domestic (formal) help**	**Nursing home care**
Spain	80.7	10.5	5.4
Portugal	73.9	13.4	10.0
Greece	71.8	11.0	0.4
Italy	59.0	29.3	1.9
Ireland	55.6	30.4	4.0
Netherlands	15.5	42.4	35.5
Denmark	10.9	46.0	32.8
Finland	17.4	58.1	17.1
Sweden	11.6	40.6	43.0

Source: Alber and Köhler (2004: 75).

increased family responsibility than younger people. It is important to note, however, that in all age groups, the proponents of increased family care usually outnumber the opponents, and in the Mediterranean countries in particular younger people are strongly in favour of extended family responsibility. In Denmark, Sweden and the Netherlands, however, the opponents of increased family responsibility outnumber the proponents even among the older age groups (Alber and Köhler 2004). It is not known whether this is the result of an age or cohort effect: if a cohort effect is at work, older people's attitudes in the future (as the currently 'young' cohorts grow older) are likely to be less oriented towards expectations of family care.

Note that the idea of making older people pay for their own care is universally unpopular in the EU countries (Table 3.3 below). Again, the 'old' EU countries are broadly speaking divided into the Mediterranean countries where the idea of family responsibility for costs is quite popular and the Nordic countries and the Netherlands where the suggestion of letting children pay for their parents' care is unpopular.

However, the myth of older persons who are not willing to shoulder the costs of their own care is challenged by the results of this survey. As Alber and Fahey (2004: 50) point out, in 27 of the 28 countries surveyed, 'shifting the burden of financing to the elderly is more popular among older than among younger respondents'. In 12 of the 15 'old' EU member states, older respondents were more reluctant to let tax payers finance the costs of their care than younger respondents. Contrary to the predictions of those who foresee a generational conflict resulting from population ageing, younger people are strikingly willing to provide care and finance it through the efforts of the economically active generation. The potential for inter-generational conflict over financing the costs of care therefore appears to be low.

Table 3.3   Perceived responsibility to pay for care of own parents, selected EU countries

	State should pay	Older people themselves should pay	Children should pay
Spain	38.1	13.1	31.9
Portugal	48.0	8.2	30.1
Greece	40.7	9.1	27.5
Italy	42.3	12.4	24.5
Ireland	47.3	6.4	18.4
Netherlands	66.2	14.1	6.9
Denmark	88.7	5.5	2.0
Finland	67.6	11.8	3.5
Sweden	81.0	8.9	2.5

Source: Alber and Köhler (2004: 78).

The positive impact of social interaction

Everybody is familiar with the stereotypical example of a recently bereaved individual who soon passes away him/herself. At the level of commonly shared images and intuitions, we therefore 'know' that social support and interaction are positive influences on health and longevity: when the support and care provided by a spouse disappears as a result of death, the remaining spouse's health can decline and he or she may soon pass away. Social epidemiology is a discipline that investigates systematically the relationship between health and the 'social' characteristics of a person's life and environment (Berkman and Kawachi 2000; Marmot and Wilkinson 2006). The progress of this discipline has been to some extent hindered by the lack of a clear definition, and a commonly agreed understanding, of the key mortality and morbidity related elements of the 'social' context of people's lives. The umbrella concept that is applied by some social epidemiologists is 'social engagement'. This term refers usually to a combination of a person's social network (individuals he or she is in contact with), the degree of social support enjoyed (having someone to talk to when feeling down, etc.) and the extent to which the person is involved in 'social' activities (i.e., belongs to a club or organization, attends religious services, etc.).

A considerable body of research indicates that social engagement or its various component parts do indeed have a positive impact on health, longevity and even survival after adverse health events such as a heart attack. Married individuals tend to live longer and remain healthier than unmarried people, although the difference is more pronounced for men than for women. Men appear to benefit more from being married than women do. Divorced men are at a particularly high risk of social isolation (due to frequent loss of contact with children, family and the lack of a network of friends) and the attendant negative consequences (greater susceptibility to illness and disability, earlier death) (Hughes and Waite 2004).

While families are of obvious importance to life in older age, it is also interesting to look at the broader field of social contacts that contains both kin and non-kin (friends, neighbours, colleagues). Approximately 25–30 percent of older people have networks consisting of five people or fewer (Wenger 1984; Antonucci and Akiyama 1987) – this could be considered the cut off point for a restricted social network. In a recent UK study, Victor et al. (2004, 2005) established that three-quarters of older people in Britain have contact with relatives at least once a week. However, it does not automatically follow that individuals with few or infrequent contacts are lonely or isolated: much depends naturally on the duration and quality of interaction, and these are harder to assess in large scale surveys. For this reason, it is very difficult (and arguably even impossible) to establish at a general population level the percentage of older people who are genuinely lonely in the sense of involuntary and enduring loneliness. Based on surveys that include loneliness modules, small percentages of the older population consider themselves lonely. Risk factors for loneliness include living alone, female gender, childlessness, great old age (75+), poverty, disability, depression and bereavement. There do not appear to be any grounds for believing that loneliness among older people has increased significantly over time (Victor et al. 2001) – ongoing longitudinal studies will help to establish the trend for the future.

Social networks: gender

Majority of those who have very poor social networks and low levels of social support in old age are women, largely because women tend to outlive their closest companions (i.e., their spouses). On the other hand, the majority of those with very extensive social networks are also women. Women's networks tend to be broader than men's in that they stretch beyond close kin: friends and other associates play a bigger role in older women's than in older men's networks (Phillipson et al. 2001). In the case of divorced older persons, evidence points in the direction of older divorced men having poor contact with their adult children, whereas for divorced women contact levels with their children are similar to or even higher than for non-divorced counterparts.

Unfortunately for many socially isolated and lonely older men, organized activities for older people such as day centres and many clubs continue to be structured around activities that women find more appealing (Arber et al. 2003). In some countries, considerable energies and creativity have gone into creating 'men friendly' social activities and settings for older men, many of whom shun the 'feminized' set up of day centres with tablecloths, flower pots, tea parties and other activities that can appear more suited for women. In Australia, for example, 'men's sheds' have been established with the view to giving men a communal setting where they can socialize through work (for many men the socially accepted and established mode of getting to know people) – with even mobile sheds being made available in more remote areas.

Conclusion

It would be foolish to deny that many older people are affected by the problems of social isolation, loneliness and lack of adequate social networks and support. However, it is also wrong to portray the historical evolution of older people's social engagement as a sad and regrettable transition from the embrace of a large and caring kinship group to complete isolation and lack of support systems. It is important to be aware of the fact that while the number of older divorced or separated people is increasing, the proportion of those who are married is now relatively high from a historical perspective, and the proportions of those who are widowed or never married have declined in many countries. As a result, in comparison with the past, similar or higher proportions of people in fact have a partner to grow old with. Similarly, despite the fall in fertility rates, the percentage of older people who have at least two children alive is in fact historically high at present, and the proportion of those who will have at least one child is set to remain high in the medium term (and possibly to increase in the longer term – future changes in fertility being impossible to predict but having the capacity to increase).

Many of the family and lifestyle changes that have taken place and are taking place currently do not have the detrimental impact on intergenerational relations and availability of care and support that they are frequently argued to have. For instance, the decline in the average number of children per woman (the fertility rate) does not necessarily translate into less contact between adult children and parents who have reached old age. As mortality has been drastically reduced, most children are still alive when their parents need help and support, and are in a perhaps better position than in the past to offer such help and support, both directly and in the form of financial assistance. Support and help flows the other way, too, with older people often making very substantial material and non-material contributions to their adult children's and grandchildren's well being, especially since thanks to improved life expectancies they are likely to co-exist with the younger generations for much longer periods of time than used to be the case in the past. For many older people, the 'personal communities' of friends and neighbours are also increasingly important. There is, in short, every reason to adopt an optimistic view of the 'social context' of growing older in modern societies.

PART TWO
HEALTH, INCOME AND WORK IN LATER LIFE

4 Health in later life

Introduction

While the majority of older people are in good health and not in need of extensive and ongoing medical treatment, the older age groups (particularly the oldest old) are significant consumers of healthcare in those countries where medical treatments are available. However, the role of population ageing in driving increases in healthcare expenditure is often exaggerated. This chapter outlines the emerging data regarding the health status of older populations, including the possible significant increases in healthy life expectancy and the attendant compression of morbidity into shorter periods of time. However, several factors might be working against the improvement of health in older age: the obesity epidemic in many developed and developing countries, for instance, is frequently cited as a development that is likely to have an adverse impact on the health of both younger and, later on, older populations. Health status at older ages must therefore be continually monitored across large and representative numbers of people in order to be able to understand the ways in which the health status of older populations is changing. The chapter also explores ageism that is often inherent in healthcare: older people are frequently assumed to be less deserving of medical treatment than younger patients, and it seems that this assumption is reflected in the treatments that are made available to them.

Longer lives: worse health?

The endemic belief that all or virtually all older people suffer from poor health is one of the central assumptions behind the argument that population ageing is unaffordable. As a result, it is assumed that the more older people there are in the population, the higher the healthcare expenditure, not to mention the related area of long term care expenditure. This argument has many flaws, however, and in order to prepare the ground for unpicking those flaws in Chapter 6 we will start by examining the health status of the older population. Are all, or a significant majority, of the increasing numbers of older people in fact suffering from poor health and in need of expensive healthcare interventions?

This question is easier to address if we first familiarize ourselves with a hypothesis (that is, a proposed explanation or pattern) called the morbidity compression hypothesis. Morbidity refers to the occurrence of disease in a population. The morbidity compression hypothesis states that as populations age, the stage at which morbidities set in is pushed into increasingly older ages and compressed into a shorter period of time. The hypothesis has an intuitive appeal. We are all familiar with images of people from the past (or indeed in some cases from present day developing countries), where they were wizened and bent over and evidently 'old' at ages as young as 40 or 50. In contrast to these images, the media is now full of pictures of strong, healthy, vigorous, powerful, vivacious and sexy people in their sixties, seventies or even older ages – just think of Mick Jagger, Jane Fonda, Sylvester Stallone and Judy Dench (these images naturally co-exist with the images of tired and wizened looking older people, making the portrayal of old age somewhat bi-polar – an observation that is further examined in Chapter 9). We are also familiar with phrases such as '50 is the new 40', '60 is the new 50' and so on. These phrases and images (and our personal experience of many supposedly older people who are in fact very 'youthful') point in the direction of old age 'starting' at a later point than in the past. Is this in fact the case?

Figure 4.1 below illustrates three possible scenarios that could be the result of population ageing. In the first case (point 1 in time), morbidity (on average) sets in at 60 and death (on average) occurs at the age of 75. As a result, the person with average longevity can expect to live for 15 years suffering from some form and some level of disease and/or disability. In scenario 2, which is in many ways the 'worst case scenario', life expectancy has increased by five years to 80, but the age at which disabilities and diseases generally set in has not been postponed: as a result, the added years are years spent in poor health – they may still be 'worth' living in some sense but at least health related 'quality of life' during this period is obviously far from optimal. In scenario 3, life expectancy has also increased to 80, but the onset of morbidity has been pushed back to 65 (in contrast to 60 at point 1 in time): as a result, people both tend to live longer *and* to get sick/disabled at a later point in time, and as a result the average time spent in poor health has not decreased. In other words, to use a somewhat worn adage, years have been added to life, but life has not been added to years. The morbidity compression hypothesis features in the final, best case, scenario: here, people can expect to live longer (on average until they are 80) *and*, crucially, they can expect to spend a shorter time affected by disease and disability that on average sets in at 70, thereby resulting in a 'morbid' period that lasts ten years and is therefore five years shorter than in the original scenario. This is also the win–win situation: older people can live longer, enjoy good health for most of this extended period of life, and therefore (crucially, from the point of view of arguments discussed in Chapter 6), will presumably both be able to remain productive and disease free for longer, resulting also in 'compressed' increases in (public) expenditure.

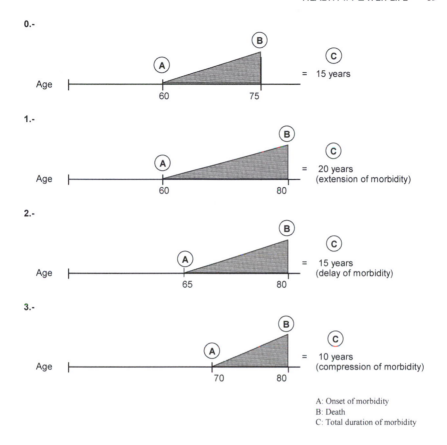

Figure 4.1 Current and possible future scenarios for longevity and morbidity

Source: Adapted from Fries (2003: 456), fig. 1.

The three main contending hypotheses regarding the changing health status of ageing populations can therefore be labelled the *compression of morbidity*, the *expansion of morbidity* and the *dynamic equilibrium* hypothesis. Much research energies have been spent in attempts to verify or falsify these hypotheses. In order to prove or disprove them one must observe population health over a long period of time, ideally across a number of different regions and countries – some of the findings produced to date are described below.

Several different terms are used in the literature to denote the period that people can expect to live in good health and without need to take recourse to significant amounts of health or social care. The terms 'disability free life expectancy' (DFLE), 'active life expectancy' and 'health expectancy' are frequently employed to differentiate between the years that the average person can expect to live without any activity limitations and the years when some activity limitations can be expected to affect quality of life and the need for health and social care interventions. The bulk of the work carried out to date on health expectancy emerges from the United States although a growing body of work emanating from European data is also becoming available.

Among the early attempts to quantify healthy life expectancy in terms of the ability to perform activities of daily living (ADL) was a study by Katz et al. (1983). From the mid-1990s onwards, researchers have been in a position to use data from multiwave longitudinal studies to provide evidence than individuals entering their later 70s in the 1990s were less functionally impaired than similar groups in the 1980s (Manton, Corder and Stallard 1997; Manton, Stallard and Corder 1997; Manton and Gu 2001) and more generally that the last 30 years of the twentieth century had witnessed a significant reduction in the rate of some types of functional decline (Cutler 2001; Freedman et al. 2002; Hubert et al. 2002). The 2002 English Longitudinal Study of Ageing (ELSA) found that 30 percent of men in their eighties described their health as excellent or very good, and another 30 percent rated their health as good. Three-quarters of individuals in their seventies were free from any ADL limitations; 72 percent of women and 80 percent of men aged 80–4 had no difficulty walking at the speed of 0.9 miles an hour (Marmot et al. 2003). It has even been argued that some 90 percent of individuals do not need assistance with ADLs or develop any significant disabilities in the course of their lives (Jacobzone 1999). Fries (2003) detected compression of morbidity in the older US population on the basis of data from the National Long-Term Care Survey and the National Health Interview Survey. However, the findings vary considerably depending on measurement, methodology and country, and it is certainly not possible to apply to all countries and all types of disability the argument that a 1 percent decline in mortality has been accompanied by a 2 percent reduction in disability over the last two to three decades (Fries 2003; Mor 2005).

It is important to be aware that the estimates of DFLE are highly dependent on the measure used. Freedman et al. (2002) point out that methodological explanations for different findings include differences in question wording, definitions of specific ADL, the inclusion or exclusion of institutionalized populations and whether the design is cross-sectional (point(s) in time) or panel-based (follow up of individuals over time). Valkonen et al. (1997) used three different measures to calculate DFLE in Finland, namely long standing illness, functional disability and poor self-rated health. While most studies employ a straightforward dichotomy between absence of disability versus presence of (some) disability, it is more illuminating to distinguish between mild/moderate and severe disabilities (Manton 1982). For instance, Perenboom et al. (2004) detected a *decline* in DFLE for both women and men aged 16–65. However, this finding resulted mainly from a rise in the years with *mild* disabilities, while the number of years with moderate and severe disabilities declined.

The support for the compression of morbidity hypothesis conceals much variation in the populations and in the impact of the diseases/disabilities studied. The most fundamental distinction can be made between prevalence of morbidities (diseases) and disabilities: whereas the former is *increasing*, the latter is *decreasing* (Crimmins 2007). Furthermore, different diseases have been shown to have different effects on mortality, hospitalization, disability and functional impairment (Verbrugge and Patrick 1995). Furthermore, the increased prevalence of some diseases (cardiovascular, osteoporosis) that has been detected over the past decades (Crimmins and Saito 2000) has not always led to an increase in disability and impaired function. For instance, early detection and treatment of cardiovascular disease has led to increased *prevalence* of cardiovascular disease but *less* disability and morbidity resulting from this condition. The effect and severity of increasing disease prevalence are reduced by healthcare, nutrition and lifestyle factors (Vita et al. 1998; Hubert et al. 2002). Better levels of education, improvements in the built environment and function enhancing medical interventions have also contributed to the reduced rate of functional decline (Cutler 2001).

Despite the evidence supporting compression of morbidity or the dynamic equilibrium, in countries that have achieved low mortality rates there is concern about possible expansion of morbidity (Gruenberg 1977). The prevalence of overweight and obesity has increased markedly in many countries: this development is best documented in the United States and shows no signs of reversal (Flegal et al. 1998, 2002). The obesity epidemic among children and middle aged cohorts is an example of a development that may result in a partial reversal in the compression of morbidity trend (Peeters et al. 2003; Lakdawalla et al. 2004; Sturm et al. 2004; Mor 2005). The increasing prevalence of severe obesity is particularly worrying as it carries considerably higher healthcare costs than moderate obesity (Andreyeva et al. 2004). As the socioeconomic status of the obese population is predominantly lower, the obesity trend is likely to exacerbate the already considerable socioeconomic inequalities in life expectancy and morbidity (see below). However, it is possible that the obesity epidemic will not affect late life functional decline adversely as the effect of obesity on mortality rates is very significant, in other words, many affected by obesity will not survive until advanced old age (Peeters et al. 2003). Conversely, individuals with healthy lifestyles and low risk behaviours (avoidance of smoking and excessive alcohol consumption, regular physical exercise, etc.) have been shown to benefit from the resulting lower levels of disability. Andrews (2001) summarizes the findings of several studies that have associated physical activity with positive mental and physical health outcomes in older age, and evidence that fitness can be regained with regular physical exercise, even in extreme old age. In the light of such findings, it is particularly regrettable that most governments continue to adopt curative rather than preventative approaches to the health (and illnesses) of the older population.

Other studies have yielded evidence against the morbidity compression hypothesis. Brønnum-Hansen (2005) studied the changes in healthy life expectancy in Denmark between 1987 and 2000. In contrast to most other surveys, the Danish surveys included older persons in institutional long term care, which lends further support to their argument that a dynamic equilibrium is evident in their results. In 1987, the life expectancy of 65-year-old men in Denmark was 14.1 years and 8.9 of these could be expected to be healthy years. In 2000, the life expectancy of Danish men was 15.0 years, 11.3 of which were disability free: in other words, disability free life expectancy had increased by 2.4 years in contrast to a considerably smaller increase (0.9 years) in total life expectancy. For 65-year-old women, total life expectancy had increased by 0.2 years and disability free life expectancy by 1.1 years during this period. As a percentage of total life expectancy, healthy life expectancy increased between 1987 and 2000 from 63.4 percent to 74.9 percent for men, and from 55.6 percent to 61.0 percent for women. However, in contrast to this expansion of disability free life expectancies, the proportion of lives spent with long standing illnesses increased: the author suggests that this reflects a decrease in severe diseases and an increase in less severe conditions, which in turn lends support to the dynamic equilibrium hypothesis (Brønnum-Hansen 2005). A study carried out in New Zealand and reported by Graham et al. (2004) also lends support to the dynamic equilibrium hypothesis as the authors detected a substantial increase in the expectation of life with moderate functional limitations.

Gender differences in health in older age

Gender differences in both mortality and levels of disability are well documented and reveal that the 'extra' years lived by women are in most cases spent in poorer health (Crimmins et al. 1996; Robine et al. 2002; Minicuci et al. 2004; Minicuci and Noale 2005). Lower DFLE among women reflects the fact that women's total life expectancy is longer and men's mortality is higher at all ages. Men enjoyed greater gains in life expectancy than women during the last quarter of the twentieth century. There has been a sharp decline in mortality from acute heart disease, and this fall has been more marked among men than among women. However, the male survivors of acute heart disease are at a risk of dependency at all ages (Janssen et al. 2004) and partly as a result of this, a convergence in the DFLE trends for males and females is expected (as a result of a decline in the DFLE for men).

Not only are there important differences in TLE and DFLE between men and women, the progression of disease and disability are also different: the progression of disability and the onset of death are faster for men than for women, which is partly the result of gender differences in diseases (Verbrugge 1989). Men are more likely to be affected by rapidly disabling, and especially lethal diseases (cardiovascular) whereas women are more frequently affected by non-fatal, chronic disabling conditions (Alzheimer's disease, arthritis, osteoporosis). Even when they are affected by the same disease, women tend to outlive men (Deeg, Portrait, and Lindeboom 2002), which testifies to their greater 'resilience to death'.

Socioeconomic inequalities in health in older age

Socioeconomic differences in life expectancy are also considerable and well documented (Guralnik et al. 1993; Valkonen et al. 1997; Jitapunkul et al. 2003). However, as Pérès et al. (2005: 225) point out, 'the important question is no longer whether inequities in life expectancy exist but rather the quality of the extra years lived'. Are the added years of life that higher socioeconomic groups experience also healthy years? Crimmins and Cambois (2003) and Doblhammer and Kytir (1998), among others, argue that higher socio-economic groups enjoy *both* higher TLE *and* higher DFLE, and that the inequality is greater with respect to DFLE. Poorer conditions in early life (as early as in the mother's womb), poorer occupational conditions and diseases linked to lifestyle and nutrition (smoking, alcohol consumption, diet, physical activity) are among the factors that contribute to this socioeconomic inequality. Better off and more highly educated people also tend to have better access to (superior) healthcare, resulting in earlier diagnosis and more effective treatments, and are more likely to follow advice on disease prevention. For example, in their study of middle aged men, Kunst et al. (1998) discovered that the higher educated men were more proactive in managing their diseases and disabilities than their counterparts with lower levels of education.

Pérès et al. (2005) carried out a fine grained analysis of DFLE in France, distinguishing between four levels of severity of disability on the basis of mobility, instrumental and basic activities of daily living[1] (see also Barberger-Gateau et al. 2000). At the age of 65, women's life expectancy was higher than men's by 4.5 years, but their DFLE was shorter than men's by 2.2 years. Inactive life expectancy (ILE) as a proportion of TLE increased dramatically with age. Irrespective of age, the period lived with severe disability remained constant at 0.7 years for men and 1.8 years for women. The more highly educated lived on average 1.3 years longer than the lower educated (at age of 65), and most importantly this extra lifespan for the more highly educated was disability free. The higher educated were less likely to experience a transit to disability (at the age of 65, their probability was 14 percent versus 17 percent for the others) and also more likely to recover from disability (29 percent probability versus 23 percent among the less highly educated).

Whereas women, on average, 'pay' for their longer life expectancies through lower quality of life, the more highly educated benefit from both *quantity* and *quality* of life as the extended life span they enjoy tends to be less affected by disability. This difference persisted even when the researchers controlled for gender, which suggests that the mechanisms involved in generating the socioeconomic inequalities are different from the mechanisms involved in generating the gender differences.

Table 4.1   Total life expectancy (TLE) and inactive life expectancy (ILE) as a % of TLE at ages 65, 75 and 85, by sex and education – the PAQUID study, 1988–98

	Total life expectancy (years)	Inactive life expectancy as % of TLE
Men		
65	16.12	20.4
75	9.52	35.8
85	4.82	62.5
Women		
65	20.67	36.3
75	12.56	56.5
85	6.76	83.4
Less highly educated		
65	17.08	34.7
75	10.22	56.3
85	5.35	84.1
More highly educated		
65	18.43	26.3
75	11.32	43.5
85	6.02	71.3

Source: Adapted from Pérès et al. (2005: 229).

Cross-country differences in health and functional status

The CLESA (Cross-national Determinants of Quality of Life and Health Services for the Elderly) project compared longitudinal data from the six participating countries/cities.[2] This study used a harmonized four-item disability measure that comprised bathing, dressing, transferring and toileting, and this measure was dichotomized into 'independent in all four activities' versus 'dependent in at least one' for the purposes of differentiating between 'independent' and 'dependent' persons (Minicuci et al. 2004). Different definitions and measurements often make cross-country comparisons of DFLE difficult or impossible: the harmonized ADL measure used in CLESA lent itself to cross-country comparisons and sociocultural explanations of the differences between the countries, which in turn are of potential use in health services planning.

Minicuci et al. (2004) found that while there is a significant positive association between age and ADL status (so that the proportion of people with difficulties with one or more ADL increases with age), the DFLE as a proportion of TLE nonetheless remained high even in the oldest age groups. Minicuci et al. (2004) also discovered significant variation in the prevalence ratios of disability across the six countries. The Netherlands had the lowest disability rates among both women and men, and Sweden had the highest total life expectancy without disability for both sexes. Italy and Spain (Leganés) had the highest prevalence of disability among men and women respectively, and Italy also had the lowest total life expectancy without disability for both men and women. Note that this was despite the fact that Italy had the longest *total* life expectancy for women aged 75: total life expectancy and DFLE are therefore not proportionately linked (as discussed above, a similar lack of a link has been established for women in many countries). In short, the results revealed a North–South gradient, with the DFLEs being considerably higher in Finland, Sweden and the Netherlands than in Italy, Spain and Israel (despite the fact that total life expectancies are longer in the Southern countries); see Table 4.2. This gradient is consistent with other research that has shown levels of disability to be higher in the Mediterranean countries than in Northern Europe and the United States (Crimmins and Saito 2001; Valderrama-Gama et al. 2002; Crimmins 2004).

Table 4.2 Disability free life expectancies as a % of total life expectancies by sex, age and country

Age	Tampere, Finland	Israel	Italy	The Netherlands	Leganés, Spain	Sweden
Men						
65	91	n/a	83	91	87	93
70	88	n/a	79	89	83	91
75	86	76	72	86	77	89
80	83	65	64	82	67	87
85	79	48	n/a	n/a	53	85
89	75	30	n/a	n/a	39	81
Women						
65	82	n/a	75	79	81	83
70	77	n/a	69	74	76	78
75	69	59	61	68	67	71
80	58	48	52	63	55	62
85	43	37	n/a	n/a	39	47
89	28	28	n/a	n/a	26	31

Note: n/a = not available.
Source: Adapted from Minicuci et al. (2004), tab. 4.

What then are the main factors that research has found to be associated with lower DFLE (aside from gender and broad socioeconomic grouping as discussed above)? Research by Gutiérrez-Fisac et al. (2000) argued that the unemployment rate and smoking were the main causes of variation in DFLE between different regions in Spain. Minicuci et al. (2004) hypothesize that socioeconomic and cultural differences underlie the North–South gradient in DFLE. In the Southern countries included in their study, the percentage of 75–84-year-old subjects with incomplete primary school education ranges from 41 to 80 percent, whereas the corresponding percentage is only 0–15 percent in the Northern countries (see also Minicuci et al. 2003). Self-reported health is also influenced by cultural and social network characteristics: Seeman et al. (1996) argued that higher levels of self-reported disability can be found in countries where help with ADL is available within the family, in other words, in more familialistic societies where informal (family) care plays a prominent role. These cultural differences may lead to underreporting of disability in the Northern countries (in particular among men who are socialized to refrain from expressions of weakness) and overreporting of disability in the Southern countries. Comparison of self-reported and more 'objective' health measurements has also shown that for the oldest old in particular these two tend to diverge so that the oldest old tend to underestimate and understate their health problems and needs.

Are older people a drain on the health services?

While increases in life expectancy have been largely driven by better nutrition (starting in the mother's womb), better early childhood health practices (e.g., immunization), improved lifestyles for some sections of the population (e.g., less smoking), less physically exhausting and hazardous jobs and better education, it is undeniable that various medical interventions have helped, and are helping to postpone death and to add disability free years to people's lives. Indeed, Freedman et al. (2002) argue that without better insights into the causes of improvements in health status among older populations (the extent of which, as we have seen in above, is in itself contentious), the direction of the causal arrows between expenditure and health status remains unclear. Health improvements may already have saved and may continue to save medical and long term care expenditure in the future. However, it is also possible that medical interventions and expenditures have been one of the primary driving forces behind better health outcomes, delay in the onset of morbidities and disabilities and less life limiting forms of disease and disability.

Older people are on average heavier consumers of healthcare than younger people (young babies excepted). In many developed countries, spending per capita on healthcare for the over sixty-fives is three to four times higher than spending on younger adults. However, the bulk of this expenditure occurs in the last year (or two) of life[3] – a fact that is also true of people who die younger. Therefore, as people live longer, costs are deferred rather than increased.

Based on the evidence for the compression of morbidity that accompanies longer lifespans and the evidence of the 'incompressible' period of morbidity of around one year preceding death, it has been argued that what matters is not the number of years from birth (i.e., chronological age) but rather the period preceding death: regardless of age, people typically need heavy services intervention during the last year of life (Steel 2005). Also, the argument has been put forward that on average the costs associated with end of life decrease with age, in other words, that the oldest old may need less intensive medical care in the period preceding death or even that they are offered less costly forms of medical care due to ageist thinking. To put it in a somewhat macabre way, at present to die older is to die cheaper.

It is perhaps surprising to note that 90-year-olds appear to need fewer healthcare services than 75-year-olds. While it is evident that healthcare costs are generally highest in the last year of life (e.g., research by Lubitz and Riley (1993), Lubitz and Prihoda (1984), Hogan et al. (2001) points in the direction of expenses in the last year of life constituting almost one-third of total Medicare expenditure), less research has been focused on factors related to lower healthcare usage (and the resulting lower expenditure). In their analysis of the relationship between Medicare costs in the last year of life and the cardiovascular risk profile earlier in life, Daviglus et al. (2005) found that a favourable risk profile was associated with lower Medicare charges (see also below).

As most people (including those at high risk of developing cardiovascular and other life threatening and resource heavy conditions) survive past the age of 65 and as the absolute number of persons in their last year of life is increasing, the expenditure on end of life care is likely to increase. However, the costs of this last year of life vary considerably depending on the risk profile of the individual. Daviglus et al. (2005) found that cardiovascular disease related and total charges during the last year of life for the low risk persons were lower by US$10,367 and US$15,318 respectively than for those with four or more unfavourable risk factors. In other words, the benefits of a lower risk profile at a younger age extend as far as the period immediately preceding death: the low risk individuals experience less disease and disability, lower acceleration in functional decline before death, and their care in the last year of life is less costly than the care of high risk individuals (see also Vita et al. 1998; Hubert et al. 2002; Daviglus et al 2003; Yan et al. 2003).

It is extremely difficult to predict the future cost of healthcare. First, as we have seen, it is very hard to predict the future health status of ageing populations. While living longer does not necessarily mean more unhealthy years for everyone, the number of people needing both expensive forms of healthcare and long term care is increasing. Second, it is impossible to predict what kind of medical inventions will be made in the future, and what the cost of these new procedures and technologies may be. For instance, a comparative analysis of dementia care in nine OECD countries (OECD 2004) presents projected prevalence rates for dementia in 2010 for populations aged 75 and over, and for the younger age groups (65–74-year-olds). The report points out that, alongside population ageing, improvements in health and social care are likely to lead to an increase in the number of people surviving into old age and therefore suffering from dementia and Alzheimer's disease. The OECD report (2004: 20) also acknowledges the difficulty of estimating the need for services for dementia/Alzheimer's disease sufferers: 'This will depend on a number of assumptions, including population ageing, availability of informal care givers, and changes in options for prevention and treatment'.

It is important to be aware of the fact that some of the costs associated with population ageing do not emerge from the wishes, demands or even the needs of older people themselves, but rather are the result of expensive interventions being used where alternative interventions would be both more desirable from the users' point of view and cheaper. The most obvious example of this is the fact that until very recently most countries lacked a specific long term care policy. Consequently, the healthcare system has in many countries been relied upon to provide care for older people who would be better placed in home-based care or institutional settings that are specifically designed to meet their needs (see also Chapters 7 and 8). Preventative approaches that could reduce overall expenditure in the long run are also very poorly developed. Infant mortality has been very successfully combated and early childhood care is in many countries very thorough, involving vaccinations, developmental check ups and even dental services. However, no similar universal, preventative approach has yet been adopted in the case of older people.

Are older people discriminated as health service users?

Supply side factors play a crucial role in determining the level of health and social care utilization. Policies and in particular the availability of services and the eligibility criteria applied clearly have a significant impact on utilization. In countries where specialized care services for older people are very under-developed or reserved for the poorest sections of the population, it can be difficult to establish the true extent of demand for services as there can be a stigma attached to service use which is very effective in putting people off seeking or using services.

Lack of screening and preventative services may result in diseases and disabilities going undiagnosed and untreated, which in turn suppresses the costs of care (at least until the time when extensive and expensive 'curative' measures become inevitable). Furthermore, treatment can be withheld or treatment options restricted on the grounds of age. In their study of the influence of age on Medicare spending, Levinsky et al. (2001: 1354) argue that 'age appears to be a key determinant in decisions about medical care for older persons'. The authors draw this conclusion on the basis of data that indicates annual medical expenditure to decrease with age. This decrease is for a large part the result of less aggressive care with increasing age. Importantly, Levinsky et al. (2001) examined both conventional and hospice care and established that 80 percent of the decline in expenditures with age is brought about by decreases in hospital expenditure and that a 30 percent decrease in hospitalizations resulted in a 50 percent decrease in the costs of hospitalization: both facts point to less aggressive treatments being made available to older patients. Care in an intensive care unit, the frequency of use of ventilators, pulmonary artery monitors and cardiac catheterization and dialysis all decreased with age, especially for those aged 85 or older.

This pattern of decreasing expenditures with increasing age cannot be explained by different causes of death. Other studies that discovered decreasing use of major surgical procedures and reduced use of intensive care units with age include Levinsky et al. (1999) and Yu et al. (2000). Investigations carried out in the course of the SUPPORT study (Hamel et al. 1996, 1999, 2000) found old age to be associated with higher rates of decisions to withhold aggressive care, even after controlling for prognosis, patient preferences, severity of illness and functional status. The SUPPORT study also indicated that many older patients prefer aggressive therapy and that this preference is often not appreciated by doctors or family members (Hamel et al. 2000). Johnson and Kramer (2000) found that at all levels of probability of survival, a significant proportion of physicians favoured treating younger patients more aggressively than older ones, even when the likelihood of survival was similar. In many countries, breast cancer screening programmes are reserved for the under-65s only, hence excluding older women whose risk of developing breast cancer is also very high. Doctors are less likely to counsel older smokers, and nicotine substitution strategies are underused in comparison with younger smokers, despite the fact that giving up smoking yields benefits at any age.

The emphasis in geriatric medicine has been slowly shifting away from compensatory approach to a curative one. It is now recognized by many geriatricians that the aim of geriatric medicine should be to assess patients and to treat treatable diseases, to rehabilitate, to minimize medications, and to resort to compensatory techniques (wheelchairs, walking frames, etc.) only when the condition cannot be fully treated and eliminated. In the future, older people themselves may effect change by become more demanding consumers of healthcare. Whereas in the past many accepted 'old age' as an ailment that cannot be cured, the emerging attitude is 'I can't run any more, so please fix my knee'. While geriatric medicine has become a central medical specialism in many countries, truly multidisciplinary geriatric medical care is still something of a rarity. A multidisciplinary team comprises physicians, nurses, physiotherapists, occupational therapists, social workers, clinical nutritionists and speech/language/swallow therapists, and is necessary for making the transition from compensatory to curative approach.

While favourable disability trends in the future could significantly mitigate the increase in healthcare and long term care costs, the increase in the absolute numbers of older people in combination with the invention of new treatments is likely to increase the total costs of health and long term care. It is naturally exceedingly difficult to make both moral and practical judgments in relation to making such possibly very expensive new treatments available. On the one hand, it seems only fair that if life prolonging treatments, operations and medicines are available, they be used to prolong the lives of older people. But what if the treatments merely prolong life (and result in large expenditure) without resulting in good, or even acceptable, quality of life? Would the resources spent in this way be better spent improving, say, childhood health, especially among underprivileged children, or in countries where children still die *en masse* as a result of malnutrition and (wholly preventable) diseases? Unfortunately, there is no 'correct' answer to these questions: individuals, elected representatives and healthcare professionals make these decisions in the light of their own moral and practical judgments and constraints.

Conclusion

Recent comparisons of healthy life expectancy across a number of countries have been summarized and analysed, among others, by Robine et al. (1999), Manton and Land (2000) and Mathers et al. (2001). There is some cross-national evidence that supports the compression of morbidity hypothesis originally proposed by Fries (2003), or the slightly more cautious dynamic equilibrium hypothesis. Many researchers have produced evidence to support either the argument that the duration of morbidity and disability have reduced even when mortality decreases, or that the proportion of life lost to *severe* disability in older age has declined. Improvements in education and lifestyles, availability of adaptive/assistive technologies and medical treatments are some of the factors behind this compression and alleviation in severity. The continuation of this trend is by no means a foregone conclusion but considerable grounds for optimism exist despite the presence of some contravening developments such as the obesity epidemic.

On the other hand, a number of particularly expensive disabilities are considerably more common among older population groups: for instance, some 3 percent of 65–74-year-old Americans have Alzheimer's disease, but the percentage suffering from this disease increases to 47 percent among the over 85-year-olds. As a result, with particularly fast increase in the number of people in the oldest old age group (see Chapter 2), the incidence and, assuming that treatments and services are available, the costs relating to these diseases are set to increase.

Older people are an important client group for health services, and they tend to use health services more than younger people (with the exception of small babies). However, the duration of the period when older people are heavy users of healthcare (period immediately preceding death) has not been increasing, but has instead been delayed as healthy life expectancy has increased in tandem with overall life expectancy. While high quality medical care is obviously of crucial importance for those who need it, the unnecessarily high costs that can arise from overly medicalized care solutions could be reduced with the use of more appropriate (and less expensive) forms of care – we will return to this topic in Chapters 7 and 8.

Notes

1   The ADL of the Katz scale (Katz et al. 1970) evaluated the ability for bathing, dressing, toileting, transferring and feeding. The IADL included telephoning, shopping, use of transport, responsibility for one's own medication and the ability to handle finances (Lawton and Brody 1969). The ability for three supplementary activities (meal preparation, housekeeping and doing laundry) was evaluated only for women. Mobility was evaluated by three activities on the Rosow scale: doing heavy work around the house, walking half a mile and moving up and down to the second floor (Rosow and Breslau 1966). Four levels of disability severity were distinguished: no disability, mild disability, moderate disability and severe disability (none = independence in each of the three scales, severe = mobility and IADL and ADL disability).

2   The six longitudinal studies are TamELSA carried out in the city of Tampere, Finland (Jylhä et al. 1992); CALAS carried out in Israel (Walter-Ginzburg et al. 2001); ILSA carried out in Italy (Maggi et al. 1994); LASA carried out in The Netherlands (Deeg, Tilburg, Smit et al. 2002); Ageing in Leganés carried out in Spain (Béland and Zunzunegui 1995a,b); and SATSA carried out in Sweden (Pedersen 1991).

3   Regardless of age, gender and education, the PAQUID project detected a *1-year 'incompressible' period lived with moderate or severe disability*. A similar

period of severely deteriorating health in the year preceding death has been detected by, among many others, Branch et al. (1991); Crimmins et al. (1996); and Guralnik et al. (1993). In practice, this period with basic ADL disability translates into a need for substantial assistance with ADL.

5 Pensions and employment: providing security in old age?

Introduction

Retirement, in the sense of an extended period of labour force withdrawal driven by wealth, not disability, and enjoyed by the bulk of the population, is a relatively new phenomenon. This chapter discusses changes in income adequacy and sources of income in old age over time and in the comparative context. Before the rise of pension systems during the nineteenth and twentieth centuries, old age was virtually synonymous with poverty for the majority of the population in the emerging industrial economies – and still is in the developing world. While the existence of pension systems and other supports has successfully reduced the incidence of absolute (and in some cases relative) poverty among older people, significant income inequalities among older people and between older people and the rest of the population persist in many countries. This chapter compares the degree of success that different countries have had in addressing poverty and inequality in old age, and draws some conclusions regarding the effectiveness of different policy tools in combating poverty in old age. The chapter describes briefly the different kinds of pension systems that are in existence in the developed and some developing countries, and the reasons behind the pension reforms that have been implemented in recent years. The shift from defined benefit to defined contributions systems and the increase in private pension provision in many countries, and the implications of these developments, are discussed.

The need to raise retirement ages and labour force participation among older workers is frequently stressed by politicians and international organizations such as the OECD. The meaning of the concept of 'active ageing' is discussed with reference to the fact that formal labour market participation is one of the many ways in which older people can make a contribution to society and the economy. The equality and gender dimensions of both pension systems and delayed retirement are briefly addressed. Modern retirement pensions evolved at a time when the external circumstances were rather different from the circumstances that prevail today, and it would therefore be unrealistic to expect pension systems to survive completely intact. However, there are still great differences between countries in how secure an old age their pension systems provide, how the mixture of retirement income sources varies, what proportion of older workers are still in employment, and so on.

Clearly, a number of very different pension systems are able to survive in a world where the 'external' economic pressures of competitiveness and globalisation are arguably very similar across countries.

Sources of income in old age

There are essentially three ways of securing livelihoods in old age. One is to 'put aside' the goods and services that are needed in future. It is possible to do this to a limited extent for instance by ensuring that one owns a comfortable home before retiring, but clearly most goods and services (food, medical operations and so on) cannot be stored for future use. The second way of trying to secure a livelihood in old age is by deferring consumption 'today' in favour of consumption 'tomorrow': this can be done by saving (e.g. for a pension), or by extracting promises from the government or one's children to provide income such as pensions in future. The third way is to carry on producing goods and services and earning an income in old age by working longer.

Box 5.1 below contains a more detailed breakdown of the main (potential) sources of income in old age. Incomes in older age can be derived from four different sources: public pensions and other benefits, private savings (including private pensions savings), employment and family and other informal sources such as charity. There has been a transition, over time and in many countries, away from a reliance on the 'older' forms of security, in other words, family and employment to more 'modern' sources, and pensions in particular. However, as will be discussed later in the chapter, many countries and social policy systems are trying to bring about a shift back to employment and private (pension) savings as the major sources of income at older ages.

Box 5.1 Different sources of income in old age

Public:
- non-contributory (universal or means-tested) pension
- contributory (social insurance) pension
- other welfare benefits payable to older people (e.g. housing allowances)

Private:
- private pension
- personal savings

Employment:
- employment/employment income

Family and other informal:
- family help/charity

It is often assumed by people in the developed countries with established pension systems that the older population derives its income exclusively from pensions. In fact, the composition of older persons' incomes varies considerably between countries: in some countries, the majority of older people derive almost all of their income from public pension systems, but in others income from employment, from private pensions or from investments makes a significant contribution to the livelihoods of the over-65 population. For this reason, it is difficult to compare the incomes of older people cross-nationally on the basis of expenditure figures relating only to public pensions: while country X may devote a relatively small proportion of its GDP to public pensions, its older population may have considerable savings or private pension incomes, hence bringing them to an income level similar to that enjoyed by older people in a country with higher public pensions expenditure. We will return to the issue of income sources in old age when we discuss the equity implications of different pension systems.

History of old age poverty

Based on his study of urban life in nineteenth century York, Benjamin Seebohm Rowntree (1901) argued that poverty is linked to age and family formation in a cyclical fashion. According to his study, children tended to live in poverty as they grew up in households with many other children but typically only one breadwinner (the father). Poverty often eased for these children when they reached the 'youth' stage of their lives and started earning an income of their own. However, by the time these young people had established their own families, they tended to be affected by poverty again as they were raising (often large numbers of) children of their own. Poverty eased again as these children gradually left home, only to increase at the onset of old age that was associated with inability to continue earning an income and the absence, at that time, of significant pension incomes.

Box 5.2 Rowntree's cycles of poverty

First poverty cycle: childhood (large families, one earner)

Poverty eased in youth when left home, earned own income

Second poverty cycle: growing family, typically one breadwinner

Empty nest phase: poverty eases

Third poverty cycle: old age (unable to work, no/inadequate pensions).

Source: Adapted from Rowntree (1901).

Old age used to be a synonym for poverty until as late as the 1960s even in the industrialized countries: the final and in many cases extreme poverty cycle identified by Rowntree was very much in evidence. While the historical evolution of old age incomes differs between countries, the developed countries share one main trend, namely the gradual increase in the importance of pensions in securing incomes in old age from the late nineteenth and early twentieth centuries. Retirement with financial security and an independent source of income used to be a privilege of a very small section of the population. Rising affluence and expansion of access to this new wealth through the creation of public pension schemes brought about the pensions revolution, and democratization of retirement. *Democratization of retirement* refers to the postwar expansion of pension schemes that opened up access to retirement in many 'Western' countries: people over a certain age gained entitlement to an income that was based solely on their age (universal), or in some countries on age and employment history (occupational) or the absence of other income (means tested). The pensions revolution brought about a situation in many countries where, on average, the living standards of the retired were no longer dramatically different from those of working age individuals.

Comparing poverty in old age across social policy systems

While the previously endemic problem of old age poverty has been alleviated (and in some cases eliminated) in the developed countries that have introduced pension systems and other income supports for older people, significant differences persist between countries in the extent to which they have tackled the problem of poverty in old age. Social policies, and first and foremost public pensions, are key causes of variation in old age poverty between countries.

In analysing poverty figures, it is necessary to bear in mind the limitations of all data on poverty. Poverty can be defined in absolute or relative terms. Most international comparative poverty research has adopted a relative definition of poverty. The Luxembourg Income Study defines households with less than 50 percent of the median income as poor, and the poverty threshold applied by Eurostat is 60 percent of the median income: everyone falling below these income levels is classified as poor. The rate of poverty in any one country or group is therefore always influenced by the definition of poverty and the chosen poverty threshold (40, 50 or 60 percent of median income). Unfortunately, even the more sophisticated measures of poverty commonly exclude assets (such as housing) and in-kind benefits such as free schemes and public services (free travel, electricity allowances, free or low cost care services, etc.), and even highly sophisticated comparative poverty data often suffers from a number of limitations such as inability to take into account the varying depths of poverty (Brady 2004).

However, acknowledging these limitations of most poverty data, analysis of poverty data does yield some interesting and relevant information about cross-national and over-time differences in old age poverty. Perhaps most strikingly, Rowntree's poverty cycles are still apparent in some developed countries, which throws the effectiveness of these countries' social policies into question. In a study by Kangas and Palme (1998), a comparison of old age poverty in the light of the 40 percent and 60 percent thresholds indicates that in the UK and Finland, pensioners had fairly strong basic security, but the level of pensions was not particularly high in relation to earned incomes. The Dutch and Swedish pension systems seemed to guarantee much better income security, in other words, prevented a significant drop in incomes upon retirement from paid work. Canada deviated from other so-called liberal welfare states in that poverty among the over-65s was low in comparison with younger age groups. Most significantly, the UK and the US remained faithful to the Rowntreean pattern where old age (and childhood) are times of relatively high poverty risk.

Interestingly, in all Anglo-Saxon countries, the (young) family phase still constitutes a serious poverty risk. This has given rise to the argument that poverty has been 'juvenilized', and even that older people have selfishly advocated and voted for policies that have taken from the young and given to the old. This view of child and old age poverty has been challenged, however, on the grounds that the definition of poverty used in some countries (including the US) is flawed. Recent poverty figures for the US also seem to indicate that the relative positions of children and older people have been reversed, and that in 2000 older people in the US were more likely to be poor than children (see, e.g., Brady 2004). Overall, however, Brady (2004: 499) concludes that 'child and elderly poverty move in concert with each other and with a country's overall level of poverty' and hence argues against the view that 'countries accomplish lower elderly poverty at the expense of higher child poverty'. In other words, countries that are serious about combating old age poverty also tend to be serious about combating childhood poverty, and countries that are less concerned with one also tend to be less bothered about the other.

These inter-country differences notwithstanding, it bears emphasizing that persistent poverty in old age is less prevalent than it has been in the past in many parts of the world. There was a virtually universal decline in poverty among older people in developed countries throughout the 20th century. In many countries the cycle of poverty has flattened out, at least for the latter (post-family) part of the lifecourse. In the OECD on average, poverty risk is higher for people of working age than for people of retirement age. The exceptions to this rule (countries where older people are more at risk of poverty than working age population) are Mexico, Turkey, Greece and Italy. Across the OECD, the mean disposable income of the 65+ population is on average three-quarters of those in working age (18–64). However, poverty among older people is more common in the US and UK than in the European states. Kangas and Palme conclude that some systems and strategies have been considerably more successful than others in eliminating poverty over the lifecycle. A study by Gruber and Wise (2002) also indicates that countries that spend more on older people do have lower poverty rates among older people.

We will now turn to examining the structure of these pension systems that have had such a dramatic impact on the incomes and well being of older people in many countries that have developed pensions systems.

Pensions: the basics

Pensions can be financed in two main ways, namely on a pay as you go (PAYG) basis or on a funded basis. The former relies on the present day working and tax paying population to finance current pension commitments: in other words, the incomes of the retired population are drawn from the taxes and other contributions (typically earnings related pensions contributions) paid by those who are not yet retired. The principle behind this arrangement is sometimes referred to as the 'generational contract': today's tax payers and workers finance the pensions of today's retired population on the expectation that tomorrow's tax payers and workers will do the same for them, and so on.

In a funded pension system everybody is supposed to finance their own retirement: everybody makes contributions towards their own retirement income during their active (working) years, and lives off the resources accumulated in this way during their retirement years. In other words, everyone effectively saves for their own retirement instead of financing other people's retirement during their working years. In reality, (public) pensions systems rarely match this model exactly: pension systems tend to involve some redistributive mechanisms even when they are based on the principle of funding. While a pension system may make the current generation of workers save for their own retirement, there is often some intra-generational redistribution so that, for instance, those who work longer pay towards the pensions of those who have shorter (or no) working careers, or those who earn more pay towards the pensions of lower earners.

The terms 'defined benefit' (DB) and 'defined contributions' (DC) refer to the basis on which the size of an individual's retirement income is decided. Both public and private pensions can be DB or DC (for instance the Swedish public pension system shifted in the 1990s from DB to DC), but the term is more often used to refer to private or occupational pension schemes. An employee who is in a DB scheme is typically entitled to a certain proportion of their earned income in retirement (e.g., two-thirds of final salary), whereas an employee in a DC scheme is only entitled to what she or he has 'put aside' for her or his own retirement, in other words, into a personalized fund that only pays out the equivalent of contributions made (and the yield to those contributions over time in the form of interest and return to investment). There is usually some element of choice (e.g. regarding the amount of savings or nature of the fund) in DC schemes but little or no choice in DB schemes. To put it simply, if Mary and John have worked for ten years and Mary has chosen to put aside 10 percent of her salary of €1000 per month, but John has only contributed 5 percent of similar salary, Mary gets a larger pension than John, provided that her fund managers have done a reasonable job at managing her pension 'savings'. In a DB scheme, both Mary and John (assuming working lives of similar lengths and at similar level of earnings) would get the same (predetermined) pension.

Box 5.3   Key to pensions abbreviations used

- PAYG = pay as you go
- funded = equivalent to 'saving'
- DB = defined benefit ('secure' income)
- DC = defined contribution ('insecure' income)

Employees tend to regard DB schemes as inherently more desirable as they in principle offer more security and predictability in retirement incomes. However, the difference between DB and DC schemes may not be as drastic as appears at first sight: this is because in many DB systems a long working history is required in order to qualify for a 'proper' (i.e., sufficiently large) pension. It is possible that a DC pension yields smaller than expected returns as a result of poor fund performance, but in principle DB schemes can experience a similar fate in the case of for instance poor actuarial projections or company bankruptcy. An important difference between DB and DC schemes lies in the extent of employer commitment: whereas employers tend to be major contributors towards DB schemes, they typically play a smaller role in making up the total contributions towards DC schemes. In many countries, perhaps most drastically in the United Kingdom, there has been a major shift away from DB and towards DC schemes among companies that perceive DB schemes to be too burdensome. The shift towards DC schemes is highly significant as it signals a shift in the burden of risk towards individuals and away from employers.

It is often argued, especially in the media and by some politicians, that PAYG pension systems are inherently problematic and should be replaced with funded systems that are more realistic and better at rewarding work and saving. As the balance between older and younger people shifts in favour of older people, it is feared that the 'burden' of financing pensions is becoming unsupportable. Similarly, it is claimed by some experts and politicians that defined benefit schemes are no longer suited to ageing societies and the competitive environment in which businesses and employers have to operate in today's world. However, both PAYG and funded systems, and DC as well as DB systems have their merits and suffer from certain problems.

1   *The main problem with PAYG systems* is that the proportion of earned incomes devoted to paying for pensions will have to increase as population ages, all other things being equal (see below for discussion of changing labour market participation among older workers).

2   *The main problem with funded pensions* is that a proportion of current resources and wealth still has to be 'stored' for future use (hence removing them from current use). The shift from a PAYG system to a funded system is also problematic as it means that one generation has to both finance current pensions *and* to save for their own retirement. Tax expenditure associated with funded private pensions tends to be highly regressive and hence of greater benefit to the better off – arguably a poor result for a programme that is supposed to secure incomes in old age. Tax expenditure on private pensions in Ireland, for instance, now exceeds the cost of both (non-contributory and contributory) state old age pension (Stewart 2005).

3   *The main problem with defined benefit schemes* is that a company may not be able to meet its commitments as the pension schemes mature. For instance, the Irish Pensions Board estimates that between 40 and 50 percent of all defined benefit schemes have estimated liabilities greater than assets. It is arguable that 'companies are inherently unsuitable institutions for providing pensions' (Wolf 2004).

4   *The main problem with defined contribution schemes* is their inadequacy and uncertainty in securing pension incomes. People's ability and willingness to contribute to pension schemes varies considerably (e.g. depending on income while working, and career breaks due to care work). The task of bringing pensioner incomes above the poverty line is left largely to voluntary private schemes and occupational schemes that strongly favour high earners and those with long careers. Funding may encourage saving for old age, but the capacity of people to save for their retirement varies dramatically. Even if contributions to a defined contribution scheme form a large part of the contributor's income and are made over a very long period, there is a risk that they will not yield a sufficient retirement income, for instance due to poor investment fund performance. The risk of insufficient contributions is particularly acute for those on low incomes and with insecure jobs. The fact that someone does not save for their retirement does not mean that he or she is irrational: they may simply not have the resources to do so. The two main determinants of pension are salary and lifetime health, and these obviously vary dramatically. In shifting the responsibility for

pensions savings away from the employer and the government to the individual there may also be an excessive belief in the ability of each generation to determine their incomes in old age: as Blake (1995: 251) points out, 'Each generation is wholly dependent on the next generation not only for the types of goods that it consumes in retirement but also for the quantity of goods that it is able to consume, since the next generation also chooses the prices of these goods'.

What aims are pension systems trying to achieve?

All pension systems are, to varying extents and with varying emphases, trying to achieve the core objectives of *adequacy* and *sustainability* (the latter is often referred to as 'affordability'). Adequacy refers to keeping pension incomes at an acceptable level: 'acceptable' is of course defined differently in different countries. In the minds of many policymakers there is something of a tension between these two core aims: the choice is often perceived and presented as being between an 'affordable' pensions system that yields small pensions and therefore results in pensioner poverty, or a relatively generous (adequate) pensions system that results in heavy fiscal pressures. Additional aims that pension systems are to varying extents striving to achieve are inter-generational equity (often linked to sustainability, especially in PAYG systems where the working population finances the bulk of the pensions of the retired population), intra-generational equity (often linked to adequacy as it is concerned with the fairness of the distribution of pension incomes across different population groups) and gender equality (many reforms have included entitlements to pension credits during periods spent caring for children or older relatives at home).

Which pension system(s) deliver greatest security in old age?

While much of the debate on pensions is focused on *inter*-generational fairness, we should not lose sight of the dramatic *intra*-generational inequalities that persist in many countries. Economic security in old age is a function of the interaction of the socioeconomic status that individuals occupy during their working lives and the pension system that has developed in a particular country. The two major defining features of pension policies that also influence their effectiveness in combating pensioner poverty are coverage (i.e., the proportion of older people entitled to pensions) and the level of pensions in relation to the general income level. The UK experience shows that universality is not enough: pensions must also be large enough to raise older people above the poverty line. Pension systems where the earnings related component plays a big role are most likely to be successful in preventing relative (as well as absolute) poverty among the older population. Germany established the first formal pension system in the world in 1889: this applied at first only to some blue collar workers, but gradually became universal. Public pensions now account for 80 percent of all retirement income in Germany. Old age poverty has been virtually eliminated: in 1998, incomes of German retirees were only 3 percent below those of employed persons on average. Recent reforms, described below, may over time erode the strong bulwark that the German pensions system has provided against relative poverty.

Foerster and Mira d'Ercole (2005) point out that public pensions are – on average and in all OECD countries – more equally distributed than disposable income of the working age population. Private capital income is far more unequally distributed than public transfers.

> On average, a little over 10% of private capital income accrues to the poorer half of older people, while more than 40% accrues to the top 10% ... On average, across OECD countries public transfers still account for almost *all* of the disposable income of the bottom 20% of the older population and close to 80% of the incomes of the middle 60% of the distribution ... Only individuals in the top fifth of the distribution enjoy a 'balanced' mix of income streams, where public transfers, private capital income, and earnings contribute about equally
> (Foerster and Mira d'Ercole 2005: 46)

Brown and Prus (2003) have argued that cross-national differences in inequality among the older population are to a large extent explained by differences in the *share of public pension benefits of total incomes* among the older population. In Sweden, where old age income inequality is very low, older people derive high proportion of their incomes from public pensions whereas in the US income inequality among older people is very high and proportion of incomes derived from public pensions is relatively low. Whereas in Sweden nearly 70 percent of incomes in households headed by a person aged 65 or over consisted of public pensions and only a little over 7 percent of incomes were derived from work, in the US earnings from work accounted for nearly 30 percent of incomes and public pensions only for less than 40 percent of incomes among older people.

It is clear that social policy in the sense of the design and generosity of (public) pensions is important for explaining both cross-national and over-time variations in poverty: countries where the right to a basic pension is based on citizenship/residence, and is complemented by earnings related pensions (such as Germany and Sweden), poverty among older people is virtually non-existent. The extent of pensioner poverty naturally depends on the poverty line that is adopted: whereas basic pension systems are often capable of preventing poverty at the 40 percent line, earnings related pensions are usually required to achieve low pensioner poverty in the light of the 60 percent line. The very considerable differences in the degree to which public pension systems compensate for previous earned incomes are shown in Table 5.1 below. Whereas the compensation level is very high in countries such as Austria, Denmark and Italy, it is extremely low for instance in Mexico, Japan, New Zealand, the United Kingdom and the United States. These differences in earnings replacement levels feed more or less directly into (relative) pensioner poverty (mitigated and influenced by the basic state pensions and private pensions provision).

Table 5.1 Net replacement rates (% of individual pre-retirement earnings) by individual earnings level in mandatory pension programmes (men), net of taxes and contributions

Country	0.5 × Average earnings	Average earnings	2 × Average earnings
OECD average	83.8	70.1	60.7
Australia	83.5	56.4	40.8
Austria	90.4	90.9	66.4
Belgium	77.3	63.0	40.7
Canada	89.2	57.4	30.8
Denmark	132.7	86.7	72.2
France	78.4	63.1	55.4
Germany	53.4	58.0	44.4
Italy	81.8	77.9	79.3
Japan	52.5	39.2	31.3
Korea	106.1	71.8	50.7
Mexico	50.3	38.3	40.0
New Zealand	81.4	41.7	23.2
United Kingdom	66.1	41.1	24.0
United States	67.4	52.4	43.2

Source: OECD (2007).

It is important to appreciate that *all* pension schemes involve the setting aside of today's resources for use tomorrow. For those who are concerned with the affordability of pensions, shift to increased private responsibility seems the answer. However, private pensions saving is in some respects not as different from pay as you go systems where the risk and responsibility is more collective: private saving amounts to foregoing consumption today for the interest of consumption at later stage: here the person foregoing (some) consumption is the same individual who will be consuming the savings at a later stage. In a PAYG system one part of the population is foregoing (some) consumption today in the expectation that the following generation of workers will similarly forego some of their consumption in the future. Privatization shifts risk and responsibility from government and employers to individuals, weakens the redistributive nature of pension schemes and fails to protect poor or disabled persons and those who happen to invest their savings poorly.

Pension systems that rely heavily on individual pensions saving tend to perpetuate inequalities that are already in existence among the population. Studies of savings behaviour show that savings to permanent income ratio rises with permanent income and does so in a sharply non-linear fashion. In other words, the behavioural response to lower mandatory pensions is a function of income level: low income families are less likely save than high income families. Pension systems that rely on individual determination to save for retirement and reward pension savings through tax breaks tend to have a regressive redistributional impact, in other words, favour the better-off, often leaving those most in need of pensions coverage with no or very poor protection. As Chapter 4 showed, poorer people (lower socioeconomic groups) also tend to die earlier than richer people, hence leaving them on average with fewer years of retirement. This means, in essence, that poorer people are cheaper for the state or other pension companies for the simple reason that they draw their pensions for a shorter time than richer individuals who tend to live longer. It is manifestly unfair that those who are already disadvantaged by their lower life expectancy are additionally disadvantaged by low incomes in old age.

Pension reforms

By and large, recent pension reforms have been more concerned with affordability than with adequacy. This means that, in many cases, they have given rise to grave concerns about the future adequacy of pensions among constituencies that are benefiting or stand to benefit from the pension system in the future. Despite the fact that pensions are a relatively new invention and a luxury that is enjoyed by a minority of the world's population, they have proved immensely popular. Due to the popularity of pensions, pension reform is almost always a protracted and politically painful process. Myles and Pierson (2001) have argued that significant reform is unlikely in the absence of a widespread social consensus among relevant social, political and economic actors. According to Myles (2002: 153) 'the political constraint on policy makers to reach reform through a "negotiated settlement" with a broad range of relevant actors makes radical demolition of the post-war retirement contract improbable'. The central reason for the resilience of pensions systems in many countries is their encompassing nature, in other words, the fact that they benefit (now or in the future) large segments of the population: where such an entitlement structure is in place, the entire population can in principle be mobilized in defence of the existing pensions system. Where the pensions system fragments people into constituencies that benefit from different component parts of the system, such defence is less likely to be successfully mounted (the prime example of this is the demolition of the state earnings related pensions (SERPS) in the UK).

The contraction of pension expenditure can take two main forms: a decrease in the number of years of retirement or a decrease in the benefits. Myles (2003) has identified three main ways of making pension systems responsive to ageing:

- *DB with a fixed replacement rate (FRR)*: pensions are a given fraction of earnings plus adjustment factor (prices/wages) – benefits drive taxes, costs of demographic change fall on contributors and their dependants.
- *Fixed contribution rate (FCR)*: working population contributes a fixed fraction of its income: taxes drive benefits – all of the costs associated with demographic ageing fall on retirees.
- *Fixed relative position (FRP)*: contributions and benefits to hold *constant* the ratio of per capita earnings to the per capita benefits. Once the ratio is fixed, the tax rate is adjusted periodically to reflect *population and productivity changes* – this allows proportional sharing of risk – *as the population ages, the tax rate rises but benefits also fall* so that both parties 'lose' at same rate. However, taxes/contributions will undoubtedly increase as a result of demographic ageing.

Pension reforms in different countries

Despite the fact that they have 'objectively' more sustainable and affordable pension systems, some English speaking countries have reformed their pensions systems extensively. Although many Nordic and continental European countries with 'expensive' pay as you go schemes face higher pension costs as their populations age, on the whole reforms in these countries cannot be described as revolutionary.

Sweden

Sweden is one of the 'oldest' countries in the world. While the Swedish pensions system (based on both basic and earnings related pensions) was highly popular, there was also a reluctance to allow major increases in contributions/taxes. In order to solve the conundrum of keeping pensions at an adequate level in the circumstances of rapidly accumulating numbers of recipients, Sweden opted to place heavy emphasis on *raising the average age of retirement*, in other words, increasing the period of time during which people contribute to the system and shortening the period of time when they withdraw pensions. Restrictions were also placed on entry to early retirement schemes.

There was also a growing recognition of the fact that the earnings related pensions system was inequitable in some respects as it favoured those with sharply progressive earnings profiles (same lifetime earnings could yield very different pensions). The *lifetime earnings* principle (effectively a DC design – see above) that was introduced in the 1990s means that earnings throughout the working life, not only towards the end of it, determine the size of pension. In another consensual move, life expectancy and economic growth factors were incorporated into the pensions formula. Provision has been made for regularly recalculating the cost of pensions, based on population ageing, and passing on some of this 'longevity risk' to retirees in the form of lower pensions. To put it simply, as older people can expect to live longer, their pensions will decline or rise more slowly than they would have under different circumstances (i.e., in the case of static or declining life expectancy). A small share of contributions is deposited in individual funded accounts. Changes in the indexation towards a greater reliance on prices rather than wages are also intended to slow down future expenditure growth.

Germany

The 1992 pension reform resulted in a change in indexation from gross to net earnings, gradual increase in retirement age, penalties for early retirement, and (in a positive move) credits for caregiving. Note that all parties, except the green party, as well as the employer and employee organizations supported this reform; they were primarily motivated by the perceived need to keep pensions contributions at a manageable level.

A further reform came to be seen as necessary as a result of unemployment and early retirement that increased contribution rates. The mid-1990s therefore saw an acceleration in the phasing in of early retirement deductions and a reduction in the credited number of years spent studying. In the 1999 pension reform, the *demographic factor* was included in the pension formula: increases in life expectancy lead to reductions in pensions (from 70 percent of average net earnings to 64 percent in 2030). The social democratic party, upon its return to power in 1998, suspended the introduction of the demographic factor and instead raised the federal grant for the scheme.

The so-called Riester (minister of labour) proposals included indexing pensions to prices (instead of net wages) in 2000 and 2001; introduction of a mandatory *private* pension pillar to be financed by *employees*. Following strong criticism especially by the then opposition Christian democrats, the Riester proposals were redrafted in 2000 and private pension pillar was no longer obligatory. However, stronger *incentives* to take out a private pension were introduced, alongside a new formula that would lead to a decline in pensions to 61 percent of average net earnings. The reform was endorsed by trade unions on condition that the decline be only to 67 percent of earnings.

France

The French trade unions have proved to be strong veto players, blocking several pension reform attempts in the 1990s. Among the French electorate, the high earnings replacement levels in the existing pension system leave very little support for private pension schemes. In 2003, (the traditionally more generous) public sector pensions were brought into line with private sector pensions, leading to a gradual harmonization and increase in the time period required for a full pension in the private and public sectors (to 40 years by 2008; to 41 years in 2012; and to 42 years in 2020).

One major union sided with the government, as it felt that there were some compensatory measures included in the reform package: improvements for those who start working at a very young age, guaranteed level of 85 percent for those on lowest wages (at least 66 percent for everybody), and flexibility in retirement age (with compensation and penalties for those who retire late/early). The restrictions in access to early exit schemes relied in part on a 'gamble on employment', in other words, the assumption that unemployment will decline and lessen the 'need' for these exit schemes.

United Kingdom

The state occupational pension (SERPS – this guaranteed a pension amounting to 25 percent of earnings during highest earning 20 years in work) was scaled back and abolished by the Thatcher government. The initial right to opt out of SERPS was accompanied with incentives for middle-class earners to take out private pensions. The cost of tax relief on private schemes took the government by surprise (in 1993, it was five times higher than had been expected). Major scandals regarding the misselling of pensions in the aftermath of the Thatcher reforms have led to tighter regulation of the pensions industry.

The privatization of pensions in the UK has led to considerable inequalities in old age incomes. Over 90 percent of those on an income of about £20,000 as against 40 percent of those on £7000 are in private or occupational schemes (1999). In 1999, the richest quintile of pensioners had incomes that were five times higher than incomes of the poorest quintile.

The low level of the state pension has created a serious adequacy problem in the UK. The state pension is increased only in line with prices, not wages, and in 2004 it amounted to only 16 percent of average industrial earnings. Despite this, the UK government has committed to reversing the 60–40 ratio that currently prevails between retirement income from the state and from private sources by 2050. The expansion in private pension provision (mainly by making private provision attractive to new groups, especially those on middle and lower incomes) is to take place alongside an expansion in the means tested pensions for the worst off. However, it is arguable that privatization has now reached the point where the central government in the UK has little control over the pension system. The new pensions components that have been introduced for people on lower incomes have tended to be little better than the minimum pension income guarantees that they would receive in any case, creating a serious incentives trap for these groups.

Pensions in developing countries

South Africa

In comparison with most other African countries (where the share of the 60+ population is around 5–7 percent), South Africa with some 7 percent of its population aged 60 or over is a relatively aged country on this continent. Pension coverage (i.e., percentage of older population with a pension entitlement) is extremely poor in many African countries. South Africa is one of only three countries in Sub-Saharan Africa that provide non-contributory pensions to their older citizens (the other two are Namibia and Botswana where the pension is both universal and flat rate). Originally intended exclusively for members of the white population (Old Age Pensions Act 1928), the non-contributory old age pension programme was extended to all races by 1944 but pension parity across races only became a reality in 1994 with the end of apartheid. The pension programme consumes 60 percent of the social security budget. A modest sum by the standards of the incomes of whites, it represents approximately 2.5 times the average income of black South Africans. The pension is generally considered to reach a high proportion of those eligible (1.7 million people receive old age pensions) and to provide many poor households with a regular income which provides a basic level of food security. The pension is means tested and black African households comprise 89 percent of those receiving old age pensions, and two-thirds of the pensions go to rural areas (May et al. 1998). Edmonds et al. (2004) highlight the effect of the South African pension on living arrangements, where it may financially enable an elderly household to take in grown children or grandchildren to provide non-tradable goods or services that significantly improve the well being of their family. It has also been found that more than 30 percent of pensions are spent on grandchildren's education – constituting a very significant inter-generational transfer (DFID 2005).

China

Until the late 1980s, China had an urban- and enterprise-based PAYG pension system covering mainly state owned enterprises (SOE) and some large collective enterprises. China started to reform the SOE-based pension system in the late 1980s. In 1991 the state council proposed the establishment of a three-tier system: a basic pension plan financed through mandatory enterprise and individual contributions, a supplementary pension plan funded by enterprises that are in sound financial condition, and individual savings. In most parts of China, however, the PAYG system as well as the notional individual accounts are still highly fragmented and publicly managed at the municipal level. The system is still in the process of transition and requires further refining to cope with the issue of financial unsustainability of the PAYG system in light of rapid population ageing. Various reform options under consideration include the modification of the existing PAYG system by raising the retirement age, extending the coverage of PAYG system to include the non-state sector and township and village enterprises, lowering benefits and strengthening contribution collection.

India

India has some 71 million people aged 65 or over, two-thirds of whom live at or just above the (absolute) poverty line (Raju 2004). As in many developing countries, retired public service workers form most members of the minority with reasonable pension entitlements. Up to 90 percent of the workforce has no pensions coverage, or only tightly means tested coverage that has the character of a benefit of last resort (basic safety net providing minimal income and food rations). State government and union territories have developed their own schemes for old age pension and the criterion of eligibility and the amount of pension allocation vary among these states (the average pension is in the region of 10 percent of average earned incomes). The percentage of older people who benefit from the old age pension scheme varies across states, from 0.3 percent to 68 percent.

The National Old Age Pension Scheme (NOAPS) was developed in the 1990s with a focus on the destitute. The national budget allocation for the NOAPS amounts to 0.6 percent as compared to 6 percent of central government revenue expended on pensions for its employees. In 1999, the central government started another social security programme called 'Annapurna Programme' for older people living in destitution. Under the programme, all older persons who are eligible for the NOAPS are given 10 kg rice/wheat monthly, free of cost: the number of beneficiaries is estimated to be 6.6 million. A national project titled OASIS (Old Age Social & Income Security, India) was commissioned as a result of growing concern for old age social and income security, in particular for the 330 million workers in the unorganized sector (including farmers, shopkeepers, professional, taxi-drivers, casual/ contract labourers, etc.). According to this project, every young worker can build up enough savings during his or her working life to serve as a shield against poverty in old age. The need for this arose because of lack of adequate instruments to enable workers in the unorganized sector to provide for their future old age.

Gender and pensions

Pension systems often maintain, reflect and even enlarge socially structured gender inequalities in the labour market and over the lifecourse. Old age poverty is more prevalent among older women than among older men. In most countries (all or part of the) pensions are calculated on the basis of salary and years worked: both tend to be lower for women than for men as a result of gendered division of paid and unpaid labour (Evandrou and Glaser 2003). As a result of low labour market participation rates among women in the past, fewer older women than men are in receipt of earnings related pensions. As women live longer than men and spend longer periods living alone in old age than men, they are more affected than men by the extra expenses that arise from run-down housing, lack of support from a spouse, increased health related expenses and the lack of economies of scale in one-person households.

In some countries, the recent reforms may worsen the position of women in retirement since the pension systems will be even more closely aligned with the labour market. The OECD (2005) highlighted that relative income poverty among older people tends to be concentrated among the very old and those living alone, most of whom are women, often widows with limited or no own pension entitlements. The risk of poverty for these groups increased in the second half of the 1990s in Australia, Denmark, Finland, Germany, Sweden, the United Kingdom and the United States. However, it must be also acknowledged that many countries have tried to acknowledge and compensate for (some of) the informal care labour that many women undertake by allocating (usually modest) pension credits for this type of work (Ruspini 1998).

Employment in ageing societies

The first part of this chapter has discussed the introduction and evolution of pension systems, and the extended periods of non-employment in later life that these pension systems have enabled in many countries. However, increasingly the reversal of this trend is being demanded: the need to delay retirement in order to make population ageing affordable is frequently stressed by politicians and international organizations such as the OECD. The EU countries, for instance, have now set themselves the target of increasing labour force participation among 55–64-year-olds from 25 to 50 percent by 2010.

We will now turn to discussing labour market participation among older workers and beyond the conventional retirement age. What proportion of older people are still in (paid) employment, and what proportion leave the workforce 'early', in other words, before the official retirement age? The meaning of the concept of 'active ageing' is discussed with reference to the fact that formal labour market participation is one of the many ways in which older people can and are making a contribution to families and communities and therefore the society and the economy (see Chapter 3). The equity and gender dimensions of delaying retirement are also flagged.

From lifelong working to early retirement?

Retirement is largely a twentieth century phenomenon: during that century, periods of 'leisure' in older age became both longer and more common following the introduction of pensions in the richer world. For instance, Laslett (1996: 179) points out that 'among the poorer people of London in the 1930s two-thirds of men in their late sixties and early seventies went out to work and brought in wages'. To exaggerate somewhat, before the introduction of modern pension systems most people either 'died with their boots on' (i.e., while still engaged in paid or unpaid labour) or retired from work only because they were so ill or disabled that continuing working was no longer possible. In other words, illness or disability, rather than the availability of a pension, used to dictate the time of retirement from customary economic activity. Within a couple of decades of the twentieth century, a dramatic shift took place in the Western countries. In the OECD on average, less than half of 55–64-year-olds are still working, and the trend has been sharply towards earlier retirement. In the 1960s, more than 70 percent of 60–64 year-olds were working in the OECD countries, whereas by the mid-1990s this percentage had fallen to under 20 percent in Belgium, Italy, France and the Netherlands, and to 35 percent in Germany. In Japan the decline was from 83 to 75 percent, and in the US from 82 to 53 percent (Gruber and Wise 2002).

In many developing countries, retirement is still not an option, for the simple reason that pensions are not available, or are so small that attempting to live on them alone is a sentence to poverty. Receiving support from the family network, or remaining in employment, are therefore the only two options that enable survival in old age. In the more developed regions of the world, some 21 percent of men and 10 percent of women aged 60 or over are economically active, whereas in the less developed countries these proportions are 50 percent and 19 percent respectively. In some developing countries, two-thirds of men over the age of 65 are still participating in the labour market (Kinsella and Velkoff 2001). The percentage of those who are making very real and valuable, albeit unaccounted contributions, to the informal and domestic economies, is likely to be considerably higher (see Chapter 3 for inter-generational transfers of domestic help and support).

It is often argued that modern pension systems in the developed countries have been 'too successful' at eliminating poverty in old age. Gruber and Wise (2002) have produced evidence that the structure of pension systems is a powerful determinant of the decision to retire. In other words, countries that offer more generous pensions that can be earned quicker encourage early exit from the labour market. The resulting implicit tax on working at older age creates a powerful disincentive to continue working. Quite simply, if it pays to stop working, people will retire earlier. The role of benefits, especially earnings related benefits, in incentivizing retirement (in the European context) has also been established by Kapteyn and De Vos (1998), among many others. Such incentives were not always as irrational as they may seem today. Governments were keen to enable early exit from the labour market because shorter life expectancies meant that pensions would not be drawn for an 'unaffordable' length of time and because retiring older workers was believed to open up employment for younger, better qualified and more productive workers.

Variation in employment rates in the developed countries

We have seen that employment rates among older people differ dramatically between the developed and developing countries. However, there are striking differences in the employment rates of older workers among the developed countries, too. The age of 65 is commonly regarded as the 'standard retirement age'. Among 65-year-old males 16 percent are working in the US, and 4 percent in continental Europe. Japan is the only rich country where people regularly work past the official retirement age: 75 percent of 60–64 year-olds Japanese males are still in employment compared to 55 percent of American and 20–40 percent of continental European males in this age group. Within Europe, too, the differences are remarkable: see Table 5.2 below. The long term trend towards early retirement has reversed itself in some countries, for instance in the US, average retirement age declined from 70 in 1950 to 62 in 1985, but has since then increased, albeit very modestly (Quinn 1999).

The European Union defines as 'seniors' or 'older workers' people who are aged 55–64 and still in the labour market. As can be seen from Table 5.2 below, the percentage of people in this age group working across the old EU member states averages at only 40 percent. This average, however, masks considerable variation: whereas less than 30 percent of people in this age group are working in Belgium and Italy, nearly 70 percent of them are still in employment in Sweden.

Table 5.2 Total employment rate among older workers (55–64), EU-15 and selected EU member states, 1992 and 2002

	1992	**2002**
EU-15	36.3	40.1
Belgium	22.2	26.6
Denmark	53.0	57.9
Germany	36.2	38.6
Greece	39.8	39.7
France	29.8	34.8
Ireland	37.9	48.1
Italy	–	28.9
Netherlands	28.7	42.3
Portugal	47.8	50.9
Sweden	67.3	68.0
UK	47.6	53.5

Source: Adapted from Fortuny and Behrendt (2002: 11), table 5.

The Lisbon Strategy set out as the strategic goal for the EU that it 'become the most competitive and dynamic knowledge-based economy in the world' (European Commission 2005). One component part of this strategy is to increase the participation of 'seniors' (55–64-year-olds) in the labour market. The Stockholm Council (2001) specified the target employment rate of 'seniors' as 50 percent by 2010 (European Commission 2005). Of the (formerly 25) EU member states, only eight are currently at or above this target level (Portugal, Cyprus, Ireland, Finland, Estonia, UK, Denmark and Sweden). While this is a diverse selection of countries, it includes no countries from Central Europe (Bismarckian/continental-corporatist) welfare states. In 2000–05, the employment rate of seniors increased in every EU country with the exception of Poland and Portugal. While the pension reforms discussed above are certainly intended to bring about this result, it is necessary to observe changes over a longer period of time in order to establish whether the trend in fact is towards higher labour market participation among older workers.

Gender differences in labour market participation in older ages are considerable within most countries, and indeed remarkable between the countries: whereas the employment rate for older males in EU-25 averages 52 percent, the percentage of older females in the labour market is only 34 percent. There is also great variance between countries when the rate is broken down by gender: among males aged 55–64, Sweden has the highest participation rate at 71.8 percent and Luxembourg the lowest at 38.3 percent. Among females in the 55–64 age group, only some 15–20 percent work in Italy, Malta, Austria, Poland, Slovenia and Slovakia, whereas the figure for Sweden is 66 percent. However, women are catching up: rate of increase 2000–05 was nearly seven percentage points for women, and five percentage points for men. Furthermore, the increase is more concentrated in the *older* group for men and in the *younger* group for women: The objective and reality of increasing female employment rates is clearly 'feeding into' the older cohorts. (In the EU, while women have moved into paid work in large numbers, the proportion of economically active men has been falling. Between 1970 and 2001 men's employment rate in the EU fell from 89 to 78 percent, while women's employment rate rose from 45 to 61 percent.)

Table 5.3 Male and female employment rates (ER) (50–64-year-olds)

	Male ER	**Female ER**	**Differential, %-point**
Belgium	52.5	29.8	22.7
Denmark	72.6	61.6	11.0
Germany	58.9	42.3	16.6
Greece	65.2	30.2	35.0
Spain	67.5	28.0	39.5
France	57.8	45.4	12.4
Ireland	71.9	38.6	33.3
Italy	56.0	26.1	29.9
Netherlands	69.2	42.5	26.7
Austria	54.8	35.1	19.7
Portugal	70.8	50.4	20.4
Finland	60.8	60.5	0.3
Sweden	76.0	72.3	3.7
UK	69.8	54.9	14.9
EU-15	62.2	41.4	20.8

Source: Adapted from EC (2003: 48), tab. 4.

In terms of the differential between older male and female participation rates, the Nordic countries form a more coherent group: both older women and older men tend to have high participation rates in these countries.

Ireland belongs to the Mediterranean family where the difference between female and male participation rates is great.

Employment rates also vary across age groups within the 'seniors' bracket: age of 60 appears to be an important threshold in terms of labour market participation.

Table 5.4 Employment rate of seniors in 2005 (%)

	50–4	55–9	60–4	65–9	55–64
EU-25	72.3	55.3	26.7	8.2	42.3
Poland	55.8	32.1	18.3	10.2	26.8
Italy	67.1	42.5	18.1	7.2	31.2
Belgium	69.3	43.3	17.0	2.5	32.1
Germany	75.1	63.2	27.8	6.3	44.9
Ireland	70.5	58.5	42.9	15.3	51.7
Sweden	83.2	79.4	56.8	14.6	68.9

Source: Adapted from Aliaga and Romans (2006: 2), tab. 1.

The level of education (a reasonable proxy for 'social class' or socio-economic status) is also an important determinant of employment rates. The disparity between the employment rates of less and higher educated grows with age: higher educated workers are better maintained in the labour force. It is also the case that individuals with lower levels of education tend to enter the labour force earlier, and it is therefore 'logical' that they also tend to leave the labour force earlier. As Chapter 4 has shown, there is a well established relationship between health and education/income (and wealth and socio-economic group): the better off and more highly educated tend to live longer and remain in better health than their poorer and less highly educated countrymen and -women (Smith et al. 1999; Marmot et al. 2003). These patterns have very important implications for pensions, for overall income, poverty and the feasibility of extending working lives. It is not fair to extend working lives if the bulk of this extension is obtained from people who are in poorer health, have lower life expectancy and will have to survive on lower incomes when they retire. The question of whether people should be made to retire later is a highly complex one and will be addressed in the final chapter of the book, which considers some of the key policy challenges that arise from population ageing.

Table 5.5 Employment rate of 55–64-year-olds by level of education, 2005

	Low	Medium	High	Ratio high–low
EU-25	30.8	43.3	61.8	2.0
Denmark	37.6	55.3	70.5	1.88
Germany	26.8	38.8	59.1	2.21
Spain	32.0	48.0	63.7	2.0
Ireland	38.5	46.9	66.7	1.73
Italy	23.6	42.3	63.9	2.71
Portugal	47.8	49.7	62.8	1.31
Sweden	57.8	67.3	79.2	1.37
UK	53.4	65.6	69.2	1.30

Source: Adapted from Aliaga and Romans (2006: 7), tab. 4.

Conclusion

In the light of the conventional poverty indicators, the problem of old age poverty has been significantly alleviated in the developed countries. Pensions have played a significant role in this progress, but considerable differences still remain between countries in the extent to which their older populations suffer from poverty. While there are many sources of income in old age, pensions, and public pensions in particular, play a very influential role in maintaining older people above the poverty line. In recent years, there have been attempts in many countries to reform pensions and to increase labour market participation rates among older people with a view to lessening expenditure on pensions and other income transfers and increasing the importance of work as a source of income in old age.

Media reports and many analyses of the 'pensions time bomb' put forward the view that drastic pension reforms are inevitable and that the affordability of pensions regimes has to become the foremost aim of policy-makers, even at the cost of adequacy. However, the fact remains that pension reform has been less than dramatic in most countries that have restructured their pension systems. There are still great differences between countries in how secure an old age their welfare systems provide, how the mixture of retirement income sources varies, what proportion of older workers are still in employment, and so on. Clearly, a number of very different pension systems are able to survive in a world where the 'external' economic pressures of competitiveness and globalization are arguably very similar across countries. Although reforming current pension systems may be necessary to contain costs, the risk that the adequacy of incomes of older people might be undermined should not be underestimated, especially for the poorer sections of society. The eradication of pensioner poverty that was achieved in many rich countries with the help of pension systems is an important achievement that should not be given up on lightly.

'Modern retirement' is likely to survive, although not intact and not without rising costs and sacrifices by some sections of society. Modern retirement pensions evolved at a time when the external circumstances were rather different from the circumstances that prevail today, and it would therefore be unrealistic to expect pension systems to survive completely intact. However, a return in the developed countries to the situation where the bulk of the population either has no coverage at all or only very modest pension coverage is not likely, and in this, admittedly more modest sense, modern retirement will survive.

6   Population ageing: an excessive burden or a manageable challenge?

Introduction

This chapter discusses the argument that population ageing poses a 'demographic time bomb' due to the unaffordable costs associated with it. The chapter provides a balanced treatment of the challenges of ageing societies, and argues that political will and pre-existing policy arrangements are significant determinants of a society's reaction to ageing. This chapter also highlights problems associated with concepts such as 'dependency ratio' that hint at the unproductiveness and costliness of older people and refers to developments that may slow down increases in costs such as morbidity compression and extensions in the disability free lifespan in many countries (see also Chapter 4). Cutbacks in entitlements for older people are often portrayed as the only or main way of addressing the growth in the costs associated with old age, but a range of alternative options have been mooted. Pronatalist policies and increased immigration are sometimes put forward as effective solutions to the 'problem' of population ageing, but their long term effectiveness in preventing population ageing is doubtful. There are, however, a number of alternative ways that can be and are being used to prepare for and deal with possible increases in expenditure in areas such as pensions and healthcare, many of which do not include cutbacks in entitlements.

Warnings about 'the demographic time bomb'

The media, policy reports and academic writing are replete with dire predictions and warnings about the growing numbers of older people and the rising cost of paying their pensions and financing their health and social care. The most famous example is perhaps a World Bank report entitled 'Averting the Old Age Crisis' (World Bank 1994). A typical newspaper or magazine article might report, in a rather worried tone, that in Europe there are currently 35 people of pensionable age for every 100 people of working age. By 2050, on current predictions, there will be 75 pensioners for every 100 workers: in Spain and Italy the ratio of pensioners to workers is predicted to be 1 : 1. As the bulk of pensions in many countries (e.g., Germany, France and Italy) are financed by the working population, increases in taxes and pension contributions appear to be necessary in order to finance the growing pensions bill. Readers of such articles are bound to ask themselves: 'Does this not constitute a cause for concern?'

Much of academic writing on the costs of population ageing can constitute fodder for alarmists, too. For instance, Gruber and Wise (2002) calculate that between 1980 and 1995, when the percentage of the 65+ population in OECD countries increased by 20 percent, spending on older people increased by 25 percent. The authors predict that if current trends hold in these countries, average spending on older persons (excluding health) as a proportion of GDP will rise from 8.2 percent today to 11.4 percent in 2050, an increase of nearly 40 percent. Gruber and Wise (2002) also calculate that OECD countries did not increase their total spending as their populations aged but simply reduced spending on younger generations. On average, they reduced spending on the 'non-elderly' by 0.33 percent for every 1 percent increase in spending on the older population. Gruber and Wise (2002: 57) conclude that 'if current trends continue, the brunt of the burden of an ageing society will be borne through reduced spending elsewhere, including spending on the non-elderly'.

We will now turn to a discussion of the reasons why population ageing is not the disaster it is often portrayed as.

Why ageing matters less than commonly thought

Countries that have aged earlier faced no imminent disaster

Wilson (2000: 9–10) points out that 'the French [pension] system was already paying out more in 1980 than was projected for the UK in 2025' and that 'although the projections indicated that the cost of pensions in the USA would be only half as much in GNP share as in France, the so-called pensions crisis has received more attention in the USA than in France'. She draws the conclusion that in debates over the costs of ageing populations, 'fear or political expediency rules, not rationality'. As Chapter 5 pointed out, concern about the future costs of pensions tends to be greater and phrased in more alarmist tones in countries that are 'objectively' facing a comparatively small pensions bill. A good example of this is Ireland where the media is constantly reporting on the 'unaffordable' future cost of pensions despite the facts that the Irish public pension system has the character of a basic safety net (being essentially flat rate and having low earnings replacement value), old age poverty is second highest in the EU, and old age dependency in Ireland in 2020 is predicted to be lower than it was in the UK, Norway and Sweden in 1990 (Fahey et al. 1998).

Problems with indicators of the 'burden' of population ageing

The projected increases in the share of the older population, the dependency ratio and the parent support ratio, the projected increases in life expectancy and the (in most cases) rather low labour force participation rates for the older population are among the statistics that are most frequently quoted in reports and media (see Table 6.1 below). They all serve to create the impression that population ageing is of a huge magnitude, and is creating a massive burden. How accurate is that impression? What do these figures actually mean?

Table 6.1   Some common indicators used in measuring population ageing and the impact of ageing, year 2000 and projections/estimates for 2025/2010

	% Share of 65+ in population, 2000 (2025)	Old age dependency ratio,* 2000 (2025)	Parent support ratio,** 2000 (2025)	Life expectancy at birth, 2000–05 (2025–30)	Labour force participation among 65+ population, 2000 (2010)
US	12.3 (18.5)	18.6 (29.3)	10.1 (11.1)	77.5 (81.1)	9.9 (9.0)
UK	15.8 (21.9)	24.1 (34.8)	11.4 (13.6)	78.2 (81.4)	5.2 (4.4)
Germany	16.4 (24.6)	24.1 (39.0)	10.3 (16.4)	78.2 (81.4)	2.3 (2.1)
Japan	17.2 (28.9)	25.2 (49.0)	8.1 (27.7)	81.5 (85.6)	22.4 (19.4)

Notes: * Old age dependency ratio = number of persons 65 years old and over per 100 persons aged 15–64 years.
** Parent support ratio = number of persons 85 years old and over per 100 persons aged 50–64 years.

Source: Adapted from United Nations (2002).

Dependency ratios

The concept of 'old age dependency' relies on the assumption that the population can be divided into dependent and productive segments. Old age dependency refers to the proportion of the population aged 65 or over in relation to the population aged 18–65. This concept assumes that everyone in the 18–65 age bracket is productive, and that everyone over 65 is unproductive and reliant on the 'working age' population. In reality, of course, some 'working age' people are very 'productive' while others are less so, and many 'dependent' people are still working or otherwise making a significant contribution to the economy and society. A more realistic measurement of the balance of productivity and dependence in the population would take the number of those who are in fact economically productive, and those who are in fact withdrawing most or all of their income from social transfers. This 'economic dependency ratio' depends critically on the trend in unemployment. However, even this measure would fail to take into account different kinds of dependence or productiveness: for instance, a homemaker's essential contribution would still remain outside this calculation, and a 90-year-old person in full time institutional care would be equated with a 65-year-old who looks after her grandchildren three days a week.

A further problem with age dependency ratios is that they assume children and older people to have more or less identical dependency levels. The resource implications of changes in the population of children (under-18-year-olds) and older people (over-65-year-olds) obviously depend on the education, employment and social welfare regime in any given country. While one country may be relatively 'generous' to families with children and less generous to older people, another may have invested more in old age pensions and services for older people, and decided to leave responsibility for the cost of raising children almost entirely to families: in the former case, a shift in the balance towards older people will lessen public expenditure whereas in the latter such a shift will lead to increased expenditure.

The potential support ratio and the parent support ratio

The potential support ratio (PSR) is another measure of 'dependence' that refers to the number of persons aged 15–64 per one older person aged 65 or older. This ratio has important implications for social security schemes, especially in systems where current workers pay the benefits of current retirees. It does, however, assume that employment rates among people aged 65 and over will not increase. More generally, defining 65 as the threshold of old age is an arbitrary convention and it would be more realistic to view that threshold as a rising boundary shifting upwards. If we take 67 or 70 as the boundary of old age, increase in the numbers of 'older people' is of lesser magnitude.

Box 6.1 Population support ratio, worldwide, 1950–2050

1950	12
2000	9
2050	4

Source: Adapted from United Nations (2002).

The parent support ratio refers to the ratio of the 85+ population to those aged 50–64, and provides an indication of the support families may need to provide to their oldest members. Globally, there were fewer than two persons aged 85 or over for every 100 persons aged 50–64 in 1950. By 2000, the ratio had increased to four per 100 and it is projected to reach 11 by 2050.

However, as Chapter 3 pointed out, it is increasingly misleading to portray adult children as the only sources of support and care in old age.

Contributions of older people

It is striking that although indicators of old age dependency and predictions of a 'demographic timebomb' are ubiquitous, the various contributions of older people to the economy and society are very rarely highlighted. In this respect, older people are treated similarly to stay at home parents and spouses whose very real economic inputs are not recorded anywhere and are only rarely acknowledged in monetary terms. Yet it is clear that many older people are highly productive in one or more of five main ways:

- *Paid work*: in many countries, the absence or low level of pensions or lifestyle preferences have forced or attracted older people to remain in or to take up paid employment in the formal or the informal economy (Chapter 5).
- *Grandparenthood*: many older people enable their children and other relatives to work outside the home and to relax by freeing them of (part of their) childcare duties (Chapter 3).
- *Other care work*: many older people are irreplaceable, yet unpaid, informal carers of their spouses and other adult members of their families (Chapters 3 and 7).
- *Voluntary work*: many voluntary sector organizations rely on the unpaid efforts of older people. Very often these services to older people are also delivered by older people.
- *Redistribution of material resources*: older people in many societies are expected to channel some of their income and/or savings to younger family members.

It is clear that we need to collect more accurate data and cultivate more positive images of older people as contributors to society and economy, rather than as a drain on resources.

Higher employment rates and overall productivity in the economy can offset costs of ageing

While the 'working age' population in the EU is predicted to fall by 20 percent between 2000 and 2050, the key factor is the balance between the economically active and inactive parts of the population. Lower unemployment in combination with higher employment rates and later retirement ages can boost the share of working population.

This is indeed the aim of so-called 'active ageing' policies that have proliferated in many countries (see Chapter 5).

Path dependence: the legacy of different policy designs

Different pension systems (and different systems of long term care) have different ramifications: for instance pension systems that rely heavily on private or funded pensions appear to impose less of a burden on the working age population than pay as you go pension systems where the people currently working finance the pensions of those who are retired (see Chapter 5). There are significant differences between countries in this area: for instance, the UK and the Netherlands have high levels of private pension provision, and their populations are predicted to remain more or less stable. In many countries, pensions expenditure will increase at a lesser rate due to various reforms that have been/will be implemented.

Economic development

There is no evidence to substantiate the commonly held belief that population ageing has a detrimental impact on the rate of economic growth so that countries with older populations have slower rates of economic growth per head than countries with younger populations. Factors other than population age structure are clearly more important in determining the rate of economic growth and productivity (Disney 1998). Future generations of older people are likely to prove avid consumers, as a result of higher incomes and changing attitudes towards saving versus consumption in older age.

Health status of older populations: needs may not increase

Chapter 4 pointed out that increased life expectancy has been associated with increased disability free life expectancy which means that the increasing numbers of older people are not necessarily translated into proportionately increased pressures on the health services. In other words, increases in the population of *older* people are not always accompanied by parallel increases in the population of *sick* or *dependent* people. Morbidity can be deferred and its duration compressed ('morbidity compression'). In other words, ageing is not always accompanied by extended periods of disability and sickness: these periods can be delayed until increasingly older age, and their duration in months or years may not increase.

However, even in countries where reduced mortality has been accompanied by static or compressed morbidity, the numerical increase in the size of the older population means that the total number of older persons who are disabled and in need of assistance is likely to increase considerably. An important moderating factor is the shift from severe to moderate disabilities (dynamic equilibrium hypothesis), supported by the findings of several research projects: the increased demand for support services may be partially offset by the shift from severe to moderate disabilities and hence shift in demand from more to less intensive forms of support. In other words, the increases in the *duration* in support required and in the *total number* of people requiring supports may be accompanied and moderated by a decrease in the *level* of support required. Box 6.2 below illustrates this possibility by outlining two different health scenarios for an expanding older population.

Box 6.2 Two illustrative health scenarios for an expanding older population

- *Scenario 1*: 20 young, 15 younger adults, 10 older adults (of these 10 all are in need of intensive health or long term care = 10 = 22% of population).
- *Scenario 2:* 10 young, 10 adults, 15 older people (of these 15 one-third are sick = 5 = 14% of the population).

Ageing is not the main driver of health expenditure

Research conducted by the OECD has shown that overall health expenditure has not been consistently linked to population ageing or indeed to any other aspect of population structure. Countries tend to spend more on health not as their populations become older, or sicker, but as their economies grow. Fahey and Fitzgerald (1997: 1) point out that '... population trends, however significant in themselves, are not major determinants of welfare expenditure – changes in the structure of the welfare system, economic development, contests between competing interest groups, and developments in policy are all likely to be more influential'. Economic growth rates and wealth (GTP) are the most influential determinants of health expenditure.

According to Eurostat, on average, within the EU, total health expenses could increase, other things being equal, by around 0.6 percent per year in real terms as a result of changes in population age structure over the next 50 years. EU Economic Policy Committee estimates that ageing-induced growth in public expenditure on health and long term care between 2000 and 2050 could be two to three percentage points of GDP. However, other estimates predict more modest expenditure growth. An analysis of the future healthcare costs by the Australian Department of Health and Aged Care (Cooper and Hagan 1999) concludes that the impact of ageing on healthcare costs will be considerable but manageable as the projected rate of increase in health costs does not exceed the projected increase in GDP: as a result, the analysis does not expect population ageing to increase healthcare costs as a proportion of national wealth. Leeson (2004) estimates that the contribution of ageing to healthcare costs varies from 0.3 to 0.8 percent of annual expenditure growth (Leeson 2004). This estimate, as well as the estimation of costs, in Visco (2001), could be characterized as being eminently manageable.

Why ageing does matter

Despite the reservations discussed above, it would be unwise to write off population ageing as unimportant for the following reasons:

Increased demand for (higher quality) services

Increases in the numbers of older people will probably have an impact in the form of increased *demand* for (higher quality) services (although such demand may not be met in all countries). Related to this is the possible increase in the acceptability of formal services. Health and social care utilization is to a very large extent influenced by factors other than the level of needs: the availability of services and stigma attached to services are key influences on the extent to which older people access services, and the resulting level of expenditure. The current utilization of services is acknowledged to be a poor indicator of the level of needs or likely future expenditure as the lack of capacity or appropriate services may mask unmet service needs. In the area of social care, stigma attached to service utilization, the (perceived) high cost of services, lack of information and lack of transport may suppress demand for services even when needs exist and are not met. The Health and Social Services for Older People (I and II) studies conducted in Ireland showed that almost one-third of the persons interviewed viewed home help and meals on wheels services as very or somewhat embarrassing (Garavan et al. 2001 and NCAOP 2005). However, it is possible that future generations of older people will find such services more acceptable and therefore seek them more readily. The extension of eligibility (particularly for free services) is likely to increase demand, and therefore expenditure, as is evidenced, for instance, by the increase in visits to the general practitioner by persons aged 70 or over who gained entitlement to free primary healthcare in Ireland in 2001.

Medical innovations and increased expectations

Medical innovations, together with increased expectations may raise costs. Whereas in the past many older people accepted the explanation that their ailments were due to 'old age', they are now more aware of the existence of cures and therapies, and are more assertive in asking for these. In all health services, a 'cure' should obviously be provided where possible, instead of merely treating the symptoms or putting in place assistive devices that compensate for the lack of treatment that would remove the cause of the complaint. Advances in medical technology and pharmaceuticals are the most unpredictable, and potentially most costly, influence on the future costs of dementia care.

Morbidity compression is not certain

Vladeck (2005: 306, 307) argues that

> projections of the future need for nursing homes and of long-term
> care more generally, or the future financial implications that such
> services might create for society are … so speculative as to be almost
> meaningless … the critical concern for future healthcare and social
> policy is not how many old people there will be but how many frail,
> disabled old people there will be, and that is simply not known,
> although the trends of the last generation give considerable grounds
> for optimism

These reservations regarding the reliability of health and social care expenditure projections are also voiced by Visco (2001) who argues that projecting
health and long term care expenditure is considerably more uncertain than
projecting pensions expenditure, as there is no framework of existing rules (as
in pension systems) that would provide the basis for estimating future
demand and supply of health and long term care. Visco uses data for 14
countries to estimate that healthcare spending as a proportion of GDP will
increase by approximately three percentage points by 2050, which could be
considered a very modest increase.

Costs will rise, but not exponentially

Lubitz et al. (1995) studied Medicare expenditures according to age at death
with a view to understanding the impact of longevity on health expenditure.
They estimated that lifetime Medicare expenditure amounted to approximately US$13,000 for those who died at the age of 65, US$56,000 for those
who died at 80 and US$66,000 for those who died at 101 or older. However,
the average annual expenditure and the costs associated with an additional
year of life *decreased* as the age at death increased. The annual Medicare
payments remain similar up to a couple of years before death, regardless of
the age at death, but the costs of care immediately before death are lower for
those who die at an older age. The total lifetime costs of Medicare increase as
the age at death increases, but show a remarkable levelling off around the age
of 80. The costs in the two years preceding death are considerably lower for
those who die at an older age. This pattern of decreasing annual medical
expenditures with age has also been detected by Gornick et al. (1993), Lubitz
and Riley (1993) and Levinsky et al. (2001). The researchers conclude that the
effect of increased *longevity* per se on Medicare expenditure is small, but the
increase in the *absolute number* of older persons will affect aggregate expenditure substantially. Other studies that present a similar argument about the

moderated impact of increased longevity include Roos et al. (1987) and Fuchs (1984).

Note, however, that this study did not include spending on non-acute medical care or spending for nursing home care. In the United States, nursing home care expenditure amounts to one-fifth of total healthcare expenditure on the older population, and this element of expenditure has a tendency to increase with age. According to Kemper and Murtaugh (1991), only 17 percent of those who died between the ages of 65 and 74 had spent some time in a nursing home, but this rose to 60 percent for those who died between the ages of 85 and 94. As a result, the long term care costs of those who live longer are likely to be higher than the long term care costs of those who die at a younger age.

Busse et al. (2002) present findings that are similar to those of Lubitz et al. (1995). Their data on hospital bed utilization provides evidence for shorter periods of morbidity before death in the older than in the younger ages: this supports both the compression of morbidity theory and the hypothesis that the average annual costs of care are lower for those who die at an older age. The hospital days data for Germany shows that the number of days spent in hospital in the last year of life was lowest for the young (24.2 days for the under-25-year-olds) and the very old (23.2 days for those aged 85 or over) and greatest for those who died between the ages of 55 and 65 (40.6 days). Whereas the aggregate lifelong number of days spent in hospital increased with age (from 55 for those who died at the age of 20 to 201 for those who died at the age of 90), the number of hospital days per year of age remained stable at 2.0–2.2 for those who died between the ages of 50 and 90. In the UK context, Dixon et al. (2004) discovered a similar pattern: the median number of days spent in hospital increased with age up to 45 years but was very stable above this age. The authors conclude that the highest proportion of acute care costs are incurred in the final year of life, regardless of the age at which this occurs. In other words, 'the total costs of acute care are greater in elderly people simply because this age group makes up a larger proportion of dying people' (Dixon et al. 2004: 4) and for this reason it is important to distinguish the costs of dying from the costs of ageing. All these studies provide evidence that healthcare utilization and the associated healthcare costs rise *proportionately*, not *exponentially*, as longevity increases.

The need to change policies and practices

Strategies for controlling the cost of end of life care have included the use of advanced directives and attempts to reduce unnecessary care (Maksoud et al. 1993; Chambers et al. 1994; Emanuel et al. 2002; Luce and Rubenfeld 2002). However, evaluation of such cost reduction strategies has shown them to be only marginally effective, one study estimating a cost reduction of 6 percent for Medicare and 3 percent for total healthcare spending at the end of life (Emanuel and Emanuel 1994). Daviglus et al. (2005) use their research findings to argue for health promotion strategies and preventive measures that could in the long run lead to reduced healthcare expenditure in the last year of life and also lower average annual healthcare expenditure at younger ages. Their

> findings underscore the importance of a comprehensive national public policy emphasizing concurrent primary prevention of all major cardiovascular risk factors from early life on as an important strategic priority for controlling healthcare costs in older ages and at the end of life.
>
> (2005: 1033)

A similar argument is made by Andrews (2001: 728), according to whom 'health and wellbeing at older ages is modifiable, and substantial gains could be made by investment in promoting health and fitness throughout life'.

Bonneux et al. (1998) examined the impact that elimination of fatal diseases may have on healthcare costs in the context of the Dutch population in the light of data relating to the year 1988. The researchers concluded that the elimination of fatal diseases (coronary heart disease, cancer, chronic obstructive lung disease) increases healthcare costs due to the medical expenses during the years of life gained. However, the elimination of non-fatal diseases (musculoskeletal diseases, cognitive decline, loss of vision or hearing) would result in major savings. This is due to the fact that while the lethal diseases caused nearly 19 percent of deaths in the study population, they accounted for only 2.7 percent of all healthcare costs, whereas non-fatal conditions such as mental disorders (including psychiatric disease and dementia) were responsible for only 0.6 percent of all deaths but accounted for 26 percent of healthcare spending. The authors contradict the popular belief that disease prevention always reduces healthcare costs (Fries et al. 1993): while acute medical costs may be prevented, the resulting long term care costs increase. Bonneux et al. conclude that instead of concentrating on fatal diseases, health promotion efforts would be better targeted at non-fatal diseases as prevention of these holds greater potential for healthcare savings.

Types of long-term care

In many countries, there is a 'welfare mix' (see Chapter 7) in long term care, and the nature, level and allocation of costs depends on the balance between informal and formal sector inputs. There is considerably more cross-country variation in long term care provision than in healthcare provision (Lundsgaard 2005). Informal versus formal service provision in the area of long term care also plays an important role in 'disguising' service needs (see Chapter 7). Where informal care plays an important role, many of the costs associated with this are unrecognized and indirect: there are clearly opportunity costs associated for carers who are not able to participate in the labour market and the impact of care giver stress on health and well being is also considerable. If (and it is a big if) the share of informal care giving out of total care giving will decrease in the future, the nature of the costs will shift from the 'opportunity costs' of informal care givers to the more readily observable and felt costs of paying the formal care givers out of public or private sources.

Within formal provision, shifts between institutional and home or community care can have an impact on costs. Bishop (1999) notes that despite an increase by two-thirds in the 75+ population in the United States during the ten-year period of 1985–95, the use of nursing home services during this period remained static. This was partly caused by a shift away from institutional and towards community care, but also by the reduction in the proportion of the oldest old who are affected by severe disabilities.

Re-allocation of resources may be needed

As youth dependency rates decline and old age dependency rates increase, there may be a case for dedicating a greater proportion of resources to older age groups.

Whereas the bulk of the costs of old age is in many countries borne by the government, the bulk of the costs of children is borne by families (although this varies considerably between welfare states). The common assumption that children are cheaper than older people takes no account of the fact that children are enormous consumers of care, whether informal (family provided) or formal (paid for) – virtually all children need round the clock care and supervision, whereas only one-fifth of older people living in the community are estimated to need some form of care. Taking into account all costs (public and private, financial and non-financial, formal and informal, education, services and incomes), children and older people require broadly similar levels of support.

It is likely that the falling number of children and increasing numbers of older people will lead to a shift in support requirements from the family to the market and the government: population ageing may have little impact on the overall level of support which is required, but it may sharply increase the share of that support which has to be provided by the government and the markets rather than the family.

However, countries that spend a lot on young people also tend to spend a lot on older people: the two spending 'categories' are therefore not mutually exclusive (Pampel 1994). Countries that have high child poverty rates also tend to have high old age (and overall) poverty rates. As Brady (2004: 20) points out, 'strategies to reduce poverty for the elderly or children should be viewed as consistent with, not contradictory, strategies to reduce poverty for the overall population'. Concerns of generational inequity have often been used as a camouflage for cutbacks policies (Marmor et al. 1997). Instead of generational cleavages, social class, power resources and political institutions are continuing to be powerful explanatory variables in explaining the politics of poverty and social spending (Brady 2003, 2004).

What are the alternative responses to population ageing?

We will now address a variety of actual and possible policy responses to population ageing. Cutbacks in entitlements for older people are often portrayed as the only or main way of addressing the costs associated with ageing populations. Cutbacks tend to be extremely unpopular, especially in systems that grant relatively generous entitlements to all workers (earnings related) or to everybody regardless of employment status, in other words, on a universal basis (see the discussion on the difficulty of reforming pensions in Chapter 5). As governments in many countries have learned, attempts to restructure pensions are usually strongly resisted by the population at large and by powerful, well organized interest groups that have in many cases defeated reform proposals or managed to convince governments to undertake less drastic reforms. Pension reforms are often possible only once their impact is obfuscated for instance through ensuring that they become effective after a very long time lag.

It is, of course, possible to take no particular action in relation to population ageing in the hope that either the solutions developed by individuals and families or the growth in the economy will generate sufficient revenue to cover future expenditure. Another very straightforward strategy would be to allow spending on older people to increase and to increase taxes and/or contributions in tandem. Governments could choose to raise spending on older people and to reduce spending in other areas (such as defence, environment, housing, education, etc.). However, such strategies might prove unpalatable to other (younger) sections of the population.

In addition to the 'obvious' alternatives of inaction, cutbacks or increases in expenditure, governments have adopted a range of actions with the view to decelerating population ageing and the associated increases in expenditure in areas such as pensions and healthcare. Pronatalist policies and increased immigration are sometimes put forward as effective and 'painless' solutions to the 'problem' of population ageing. The following discussion focuses on some of these 'painless' policy responses that do not require any sacrifices by younger or older population groups.

Box 6.3 What can be done about population ageing and its consequences?

1 Encouraging more childbearing (*pronatalism*).
2 Public *health promotion* measures.
3 Promoting *immigration* of working age people.
4 *Reforming* social policy (e.g., higher retirement age).
5 *Cutbacks* in entitlements, rationing treatments.
6 Enhancing *productivity* and *labour market* participation (expansion of other 'reserve' workforce components – e.g., women).

Pronatalism

Pronatalism refers to policies that seek to make childrearing more financially or practically manageable. The intention is to use policy-based incentives to persuade people to have more children in order to 'generate' more young (and hopefully eventually productive) people in the population.

Fertility decline can be slowed down with the help of appropriate policies under some circumstances (RAND Europe 2005). For instance, pronatalism in France (childcare subsidies, rewards for having three or more children) has resulted in the second highest fertility rate in Europe (after Ireland with its negligible degree of pronatalism!) and even an increase in the fertility rate in 1993–2002. However, there is no single universally successful 'trick' to halt or reverse fertility decline. In Sweden, flexible working and generous parental leave entitlements had (the largely unintended) by-product of increased fertility. The social, political and economic contexts of policy interventions also influence outcomes. Eastern Germany and Poland saw declines in fertility following the 1989 fall of communism and the instability that followed in its wake. Conversely, improvements in social and economic conditions *may* lead to improvements in fertility. The long time lags associated with the pronatalist strategy are unattractive for politicians – there is an obvious disparity between the short time cycles of politics (typically four to five years between elections) and the much longer time cycles of fertility (two decades or more before increased births feed into the labour force). Furthermore, a change in the timing of births (bringing them forward) is no good if completed (total) fertility does not increase.

Investment in healthy and active ageing

The research discussed in Chapter 4 shows that the onset of chronic disease associated with old age and accompanying disability can be delayed, and that health promotion and prevention of diseases in old age can be effective. Chapter 5 highlighted the fact that enabling more people to work longer can dramatically reduce the number of people drawing all or most of their income from pensions. However, these strategies are obviously long term, and require investing in education and preventative healthcare and as such are not particularly appealing to politicians who operate within shorter time frames and have a tendency to focus on acute crises rather than on long term strategies that may yield benefits decades from now.

Immigration

Increased immigration is sometimes put forward as an 'instant solution' to population ageing. This suggestion assumes that the immigrants will be of working age, that they will be able to slot into jobs and that (as an additional boon) their fertility levels will be higher than those in the 'indigenous' population. However, the OECD has estimated that immigration might have to be between five and ten times its current level in order to neutralize the effects of ageing populations. Unfortunately, based on past experience, many societies find it hard to accept such large numbers of immigrants. Obviously, the immigrants will eventually age, and at least the first generation of immigrants, upon retiring, would be disproportionately likely to be poor and hence in need of extensive support. Immigrants also tend to adopt their host country's fertility behaviour (i.e., typically they have fewer children than they would have had in their country of origin), which necessitates successive waves of new immigrants if the balance between working age and retired people is to be maintained with the help of the immigration method.

Shift from 'more expensive' to 'cheaper' forms of care

In order to control expenditure, governments would be well advised to invest more in community care and innovative supports for home-based care, instead of in institutional care. However, this route to slowing expenditure growth has its limits, and its feasibility depends on a number of variables, especially the availability of informal care that typically underpins community care even where extensive formal services are made available (see Chapters 7 and 8).

Reform of social policy

Reforming social policies by for instance cutting back pension entitlements (or making it harder to achieve expected levels of entitlements) appears justified in the light of increased life expectancy and better health among the older population. It also appears desirable due to the expected exchequer savings. Indeed, as Chapter 10 argues, policies that incentivize longer working lives could even be construed as anti-ageist as one of the results would be lessened dependency of the older population on social welfare and their greater engagement in the active and socially valued sphere of paid employment. However, as Chapter 10 argues, such a strategy requires several enabling policies and needs to be mindful of socioeconomic and gender inequalities in life expectancy, careers and pay if it is to be implemented in a fair way.

The negative aspects of such reforms are also apparent, and are discussed in a number of chapters in this book. Reforms that tamper with entitlements tend to be extremely unpopular, not only among the older but also younger population groups where they have a realistic expectation of benefiting from the entitlements in the future. Such reforms can also hit the wrong groups, in other words, those who need assistance most. Even where they are implemented, reforms in the area of pensions can have very long time lags – it often takes several decades for the impact of pension reform to become manifest. Today's politicians may therefore be reluctant to take the pain of their electorate's displeasure for gain in the future when they may no longer be in office.

Enhancing productivity: labour market participation

One 'obvious' source of reserve labour is women. The problem with this strategy is that it places great demands on women, especially if combined with a drive to increase fertility. This policy seems to suggest that women have to do everything – have babies *and* work more (or, alternatively, that some women should 'specialize' in reproduction and others in economic production – also a rather unpalatable concept). In order to maximize the chances of success, the ambition to both raise fertility and increase female labour market participation levels should be backed up with increased supports for families with children (childcare, income transfers), for working mothers (childcare, employment rights, equal opportunities) and also with attempts to alter the traditional distribution of care work and domestic labour between men and women.

While some countries (notably France and the Nordic countries) have managed to induce more women to both reproduce at a comparative high rate and to work, it is not certain that a similar strategy would work in all other countries, or that it will continue to work. It is to be hoped that any policies that try to incentivize women to adopt dual roles would extend such incentives to men, or indeed make the receipt of benefits and supports conditional on men (fathers) doing their share of the domestic and childrearing duties that still have to be completed in dual earner households.

Conclusion

How much does ageing really matter? This is not an easy question to answer; indeed there is a case for arguing that it is impossible to know the answer due to the large number of highly uncertain variables involved. Much depends both on the extent of emerging and changing needs among older people, and on the ability or willingness of the society and governments to respond to these needs. There are a large number of micro and macro level factors that determine this. The key variables are the healthcare needs of older people (possibly getting healthier – morbidity compression – but possibly not), older people's expectations about the amount and quality of services they wish to receive, labour market participation among women and other factors that are related to families' willingness to offer unpaid care. Economic growth, productivity, changes in the labour force, welfare state structures (whether public or private provision dominates, whether pensions are PAYG or funded, whether community or institutional care is given primacy) are also highly influential. So far no consensus has emerged on the exact impact of population ageing, and given the large number of uncertain variables, predicting the costs in the long term yields highly uncertain estimates.

However, it is certainly wrong to portray population ageing as a crisis or a threat. Ageing should be seen as a great achievement that requires re-adjustment in policies and attitudes, but is fundamentally a positive development that can yield benefits not only to older people in the form of longer and healthier lives but also to younger generations in the form of the many different contributions that older people make.

Population ageing, which is a universal and ongoing phenomenon, has generated much concern about the accompanying costs in the areas of healthcare and social (long term) care. The clear majority of studies focusing on the determinants of overall healthcare expenditure have identified (national) income, lifestyles and environmental factors as the key determinants of expenditure: the age structure of the population does not seem to be a very strong explanatory factor in comparison with the other factors (Jacobzone 1999). Despite this, a very large volume of research has investigated the relationship between age and healthcare use, and the related healthcare expenditure. Although analyses of healthcare expenditure have revealed a relationship between age, health status and related expenditure, this relationship is very complex. Most importantly, researchers have established that a very large proportion of the increased expenditure in older age groups takes place during the year preceding death, and a similar pattern exists for persons who die before entering old age: the last year of life has considerable resource implications, regardless of the age at which death occurs. It is therefore possible to conclude that healthcare expenditure is not so much related to age as to the proximity of death. Moreover, there is much variance in the expenditure during the final year depending on health status as the cost of care for individuals with low risk behaviours tends to be lower.

All calculations regarding the expenditure implications of population ageing are highly uncertain and provisional, chiefly because age specific care utilization patterns change over time. Moreover, with the development of specific long term care policies and services in many (although not all) countries, the expenditure that is relevant for the oldest age groups is increasingly 'social' (long term) care expenditure, rather than healthcare expenditure. To date very few attempts have been made to estimate the future long term care costs and indeed these attempts are curtailed by the uncertainty related to the level of future care needs, the availability of informal care, innovations in medical care, pharmaceuticals and assistive devices, and the future trajectory of policy development (e.g., a shift from institutional to domiciliary care could have major repercussions on the costs of care).

It is evident that different countries invest very different amounts in social protection of older people: while some are very high spenders, others rely on individual and family contributions to care and incomes in old age. It is also evident that the high spenders have not suffered the dire consequences that population ageing is often argued to bring: it is evidently feasible, where the political will and popular support exist, to spend heavily on the old age population *and* to have a successful economy with high employment rates, *and* to invest in younger age groups.

PART THREE
CARE OF OLDER PERSONS

7 Care services for older people I: informal and formal

Introduction

The area of long term care for older people is a highly complex one. This chapter sets out the basic conceptual and analytical tools that are necessary for making sense of long term care services for older people. The difference between formal and informal services is highlighted; the possible and increasingly common separation of provider and purchaser functions is discussed; and the extent of formal service provision in different countries is compared. The chapter also describes recent changes in long term care policies in a number of countries and discusses the use of 'social care regimes' in simplifying the often very complex reality of long term care.

Defining 'care'

Clearly, the term 'care' is multifaceted, as it relates to both health (medical/paramedical) and social care. Medical care, despite its complexities, is nonetheless reasonably easily defined as attempts to cure or alleviate physical or mental illness. Chapter 6 has already alerted the reader to the fact that long term care is highly, and arguably unnecessarily, 'medicalized' in many countries, and that health services and medicines are often deployed where 'social' services and rehabilitative interventions would be more appropriate. What, then, are the *non-medical* elements of long term care?

The OECD (2005: 10) defines long term care as:

> ...a range of services for persons who are dependent on help with basic activities of daily living (ADL) over an extended period of time. Such activities include bathing, dressing, eating, getting in and out of bed or chair, moving around and using the bathroom. These long-term care needs are due to long-standing chronic conditions causing physical or mental disability.

The term 'social or long term care' can also be used in a wider sense to denote assistance not only activities of daily living (ADL) as specified above, but also assistance with instrumental activities of daily living (IADL), in other words, domestic work such as cleaning and cooking, and other basic day to day 'life management' tasks such as paying bills, shopping, running errands, and so on. The definition of long term care can also include 'light touch' services such as supervision (for instance of a person with dementia who is liable to wander and put him/herself at a risk that is deemed unacceptably high) or purely 'social' aspects such as companionship. Health and the more 'social' forms of care are naturally inter-linked, although policies and institutions are not always able to ensure that these two types of care are provided in tandem or interchangeably. For instance, an older person may need to stay in hospital for a period when undergoing an operation or recuperating from a serious illness. Upon discharge from hospital, a combination of medical and social services may be required to enable the older person to return to the home environment: indeed the availability of such community-based services (and/or informal family care) is often a prerequisite of safe and successful hospital discharge.

Chapters 4 and 6 have already noted, but it is worth emphasizing, that the clear majority of older people are *not* in any need of care. For instance, before the age of 80, less than 10 percent of older Germans require care, after which the percentage increases to roughly one-quarter among those aged 85–9, still a remarkably low percentage (Alber and Schölkopf 1999). In the UK, the estimated *lifetime* risk of (ever) needing residential care for a woman aged 65 is 36 percent, and for a man of this age 20 percent (Department of Social and Family Affairs 2002). Nonetheless, for those older people who do require care, the availability, location, cost and quality of care are of great importance.

One of the striking things about 'care' is that while it is obviously ubiquitous, we know very little about it. Why is this the case? The central explanation lies in the fact that much of care work takes place in the private sphere, behind closed doors, outside the formal economy and is not accounted for in ways that most other types of work are (in employment, GDP, productivity, etc., statistics). Wærness (1978) coined a very appropriate term, that of 'an invisible welfare state of care' which reflects the neglect of care in statistics, welfare regime classifications, and often even in public debates on 'important' social policy issues. For those who need help and care, family is the most common source of assistance virtually everywhere, with the possible exception of some Nordic countries. Despite this commonality, the exact division of responsibility for the care of older people varies enormously between parts of the world and individual countries. We will now turn to analysing the different sources, or providers, of long term care for older people.

Who provides care? The informal/formal care distinction

Long term care is received in many different settings, and is carried out by a wide range of carers ranging from medical 'professionals' to 'formal' (paid) carers to 'informal' or family carers (who in most cases are not paid but can receive various benefits and subsidies from the government – see under 'who finances care?'). *Informal* care can also be referred to as *family* or *unpaid* care, denoting the fact that it is delivered by family members, neighbours or friends, typically in the recipient's or carer's home, usually without any financial recompense. *Formal* or *paid* care, on the other hand, can be provided either in the community (in the older person's home or in a public community setting such as a daycare centre) or in a residential institution (home, community and institutional care are discussed in greater detail in Chapter 8).

A complex 'care mix' exists in many countries that have both formal and informal care services operating in parallel (of course, many countries continue to rely exclusively, or almost exclusively, on informal care and have not developed the formal care services sector). The actors involved in the provision of *formal* care can be drawn from the public (government), private (for profit) or voluntary (non-profit or charitable) sectors. Table 7.1 below illustrates these basic distinctions. However, it is essential to note that the boundary between formal and informal is becoming increasingly fuzzy as governments make payments to facilitate and encourage informal care, and the boundary between the public and private sectors is also blurred as payments from the government are increasingly used to purchase care from private (profit-making) providers in many countries (Fine 2007).

The European Observatory on Ageing and Older People reported in 2003 that with the exception of Denmark, all Western European countries rely on families to provide the bulk of care. Tester (1996) estimates that the share of informal care of all care is around 75–80 percent. OECD (1996) has also estimated that across countries around three-quarters of the sum total of care for frail older persons is provided by informal carers. Even in countries where extensive public or private care services are available, informal carers often perform an essential 'care management' role that enhances the integration of the otherwise fragmented structures of service provision. Nonetheless, we know remarkably little about even the most basic aspects of informal care such as its quantity, agency, and cost (direct and opportunity cost).

In the Nordic countries the introduction of public childcare and elder care services in the post-Second World War period was one of factors that contributed to and enabled the rapidly rising labour market participation among women. In many of the countries that have not to date developed such public care services, population ageing, changes in family structures and living arrangements of older persons, in combination with changes in

Table 7.1 Informal and formal care

Provider	Informal ('family') carer	Formal ('paid') carer		
Location	Usually the care recipient's own home (although in some cases move into care giver's home takes place; some types of informal care can also be given in an institutional or residential setting, especially where staff shortages mean that residential care has to be supplemented by family members who, e.g., bring in meals).	Care recipient's home ('domiciliary care').	Community setting such as a daycare centre.	Institution (nursing home or similar).
Carer	Family member, friend, neighbour who is usually unpaid, but see below.	Care workers can be employed by the public, private or non-profit sectors. In some countries, some paid care workers in the home have no formal anchoring to an employer and no formal status (they are operating in the 'grey' labour market).		
Financing	De facto usually the informal care giver ('opportunity cost'); in some cases an informal carer is in receipt of a subsidy from the government (carer's allowance, long term care insurance payment for an informal carer or similar).	Continuum from completely private financing to full coverage of costs by the government (see below under who pays for care).		

women's lifestyles, are leading to an increased demand for formal (public and private) care services. This does not mean, however, that the importance of informal care is being seriously eroded: family care is also continuing to expand in tandem with formal service provision, although in some cases family care is being oriented more towards companionship and away from 'heavy duty' assistance with activities of daily living.

Who are the informal (family) carers?

The situation and profile of carers varies greatly depending on the number of hours per week that they spend caring, the level of care needs of the person they care for, the carers' own health, and so on. It is correct to state, however, that (1) most 'heavy duty' carers are female; (2) the great majority of 'heavy duty' carers are not engaged in paid work (i.e., work outside the informal care they perform); and (3) that they suffer disproportionately from poverty due to the loss of opportunities to engage in paid work and the greater propensity of lower income individuals to become involved in full time informal care work.

According to a recent survey (Alber and Köhler 2004), approximately one-fifth of the citizens of the EU-15 member states are regularly providing informal help and care to other people living with them or outside their own household.[1] Focusing on older people (defined here as aged 60 and over) as care recipients, it is interesting to note that informal care provision to older people is widespread in many countries that offer a high level of formal services, too (Alber and Köhler 2004). To simplify somewhat, it appears that informal care is more common in South than in North Europe (and also more common in the new member states in the 'East' than in the old member states in the 'West'), although this divide becomes blurred in the case of services provided to people outside the household. While informal care provision to someone outside the household is comparatively rare in the Mediterranean countries, care provision to someone in the household (a co-resident) is more common in these countries than in the EU-15 on average (Alber and Köhler 2004). The rarity of multigenerational households is the main reason behind the low proportion of Nordic and Dutch people providing care within private households (see also Chapter 3). The provision of formal services does not appear to crowd out informal help; in fact, the opposite would seem to be the case in a number of countries with highly developed care services (e.g., Netherlands, Finland, Sweden). In these cases, a 'division of labour' emerges between the formal providers who deliver assistance with activities of daily living and family members who provide companionship and assistance with domestic tasks (Motel-Klingebiel et al. 2005).

Perhaps somewhat surprisingly, the survey results indicate that roughly similar proportions of women (23 percent) and men (21 percent) are providing informal care. While there are a number of reasons for this result, the fact that the informal care input is not disaggregated by the nature of the care work performed (e.g., personal care such as bathing is obviously radically different from many household tasks such as shopping or garden maintenance) or the time devoted to care work (e.g., full time care work versus checking on someone once or twice a week) is a serious shortcoming of this and many other studies.

The probability of being an informal carer peaks in middle age, and amounts of care do not differ significantly among the employed, unemployed or retired individuals. This means, as Alber and Fahey (2004: 49) point out, that 'people outside the labour force do not effectively lower the burden for working people who frequently have to juggle work and caring roles'. The dual pressures of work and care often result in high levels of stress and disruption of both family life and career, especially in the case of people who are caring for both older relatives and their own children (Phillips et al. 2002; see also Chapter 3).

Formal care services

Unfortunately, in assessing the extent and nature of formal services across countries we only have rather limited information at our disposal. These limitations in the available information are partly due to the nature of the care sector. The formal care services sector is a messy area of research as a result of, among other factors, usually decentralized service delivery, lack of (comprehensive) statistics, and the difficulty in some cases of separating health and social services. The government can facilitate care of older people in two main ways: it can either *provide* services directly or it can help individuals to *finance* (all or part of) the cost of services that are purchased from other providers. In order to gauge the extent of government responsibility, we therefore need to take into account both the extent of direct service provision and the extent of financial support specifically targeted at care (instead of general income maintenance). Second, the informal ('grey') economy of care appears to play a growing role in this area. It is exceedingly difficult to assess the extent of care provision in the grey market or the resources devoted to such provision by individuals. Third, in all areas of provision and in most countries, statistics are incomplete and have to be treated with caution. Most statistics relate to public provision and financing only, leaving out or providing only very approximate estimates of private expenditure on care.

A more detailed discussion of formal care services is contained in Chapter 8. Here, we merely highlight the differences in the extent to which the government is involved in financing care in a small number of selected countries. Public long term care expenditure is comparatively extensive in Germany, Japan and Sweden. Within this group of relatively high spenders, differences are considerable: the nearly 3 percent invested in Sweden is considerably higher than expenditure in the next highest spender, Germany. In long term care systems that depend in part or wholly on means testing, public spending is typically lower. In most countries, public outweighs private expenditure: exceptions tend to be countries where public provision and subsidies are negligible and any formal care must be privately purchased (e.g., Spain). It is important here to bear in mind the precaution highlighted above, namely that any statistics on purely private long term care spending are imperfect or lacking in most countries.

Table 7.2 Public and private expenditure on long term care, % of GDP, 2000

Country	Total	Public	Private
OECD average	1.25	0.99	0.24
Australia	1.19	0.86	0.33
Canada	1.23	0.99	0.24
Germany	1.35	0.95	0.40
Japan	0.83	0.76	0.07
Spain	0.61	0.16	0.44
Sweden	2.89	2.74	0.14
United States	1.29	0.74	0.54

Source: OECD (2005).

Gender dimension of informal and formal care

It has been estimated that seven out of ten men are married or living with someone when they die, whereas seven out of ten women are living alone when they die. Largely as a result of gender differences in disability and the numerical imbalance of men and women in later life (see Chapters 2 and 4), the provision and receipt of informal care are gendered. Women are less likely than men to have a spouse to provide care and enable them to live in the community at the later stages of their lives when they are most likely to need care. Whereas most men die married, in other words, they can rely on wives to provide care, older women (whose predominant status at death is widow) have to call upon their children or formal home care providers or go into residential care. Partly due to this pattern and to the smaller number of male informal carers, attitudes towards male and female carers also vary considerably. Whereas male carers are often perceived as extraordinary heroes (many of them obviously deservedly so), female carers are usually (unfairly) taken for granted.

Interestingly, the gendered pattern of care is evident in the sphere of *formal* services, too. In Sweden, a country noted for its extensive formal care provision, approximately 90 percent of staff in municipal (public sector) care for older people and 95 percent of the supervisors/managers in this sector are women. Statistics Sweden (2000) established that there are 700,000 workers in the social and care sector, equivalent to 20 percent of all employees in the Swedish labour market. Thirty-five percent of all female employees and 5 percent of all male employees in Sweden work in this sector. Note also that, on average, wages in the private sector in 2001 in Sweden were approximately 14 percent higher than in the public sector. Even in a highly developed 'service state', care work tends to be gendered and low paid. Very different care regimes can therefore mask the rather similar divisions of the overall care labour between women and men: countries that rely overwhelmingly on families to provide care are drawing on women's informal care work, but countries that have highly developed formal care provision also rely on women as they constitute the bulk of employees in this sector.

To what extent should families be responsible for older people?

Who *should* be responsible for providing the care that some older people need? This is one of the most controversial topics of normative debate among students of ageing, policymakers and indeed the general public. In some societies, families are assumed to shoulder full responsibility. In others, the government is seen as the primary provider. The underlying and ensuing differences in how care is thought of and delivered are considerable.

A number of thorny issues naturally ensue on both sides of the argument. Those who argue that families should provide care are called upon to specify what exactly they mean by 'family': adult children, spouses, more distant relations? Should and can the responsibility for caring be shared between several family members, male and female? What about people who have no family, or who have only a very small family, or family members who are all working and have young children to look after? Those who adopt the opposite stance and argue that care should be primarily the responsibility of the government also have to answer a number of difficult questions. Who exactly is to finance this care? How do we know that the care will be of good quality? Does welfare state involvement in the form of more services crowd out family involvement?

While 'principal care givers' may be receiving help from others, such help usually amounts to a very small fraction of the input of the principal carer (Hughes et al. 2005). Informal care is, therefore, in most cases shouldered by single individuals, many of whom work up to and in excess of 100 hours per week performing different care duties (physical and household care, supervision, companionship, administration of medicines and paperwork, etc.). Unfortunately, working time directives and many other protections do not apply to these carers whose work is also often financially and otherwise unrecognized.

A number of questions arise here. First, to what extent is such care work purely *voluntary*? A rough indicator of the 'genuine willingness' of people to provide informal care may be in their preferences regarding the possibility of re-inforcing the duty to care for older relatives. The results of a survey will be discussed below to shed light on this. Second, regardless of whether it is voluntary or not, is it *fair* or *reasonable* to expect people to perform such intensive care work without compensation and support? Third, will the growth in the demand for care outstrip the supply of informal care, thus exposing older people to the risk of unmet care needs if we continue to rely on informal care? Fourth, in the light of the answers to the three questions posed above, is it appropriate to put in place policies that facilitate the substitution of formal for informal care?

With regard to the question of voluntary or involuntary nature of informal care, it is in practice impossible to tell what proportion of informal care work is truly voluntary. Research on carers has indicated that informal carers often 'drift' into their role (Begley and Cahill 2003). The carer may initially be providing help one or two hours a day, but when care needs increase they gradually or suddenly become more involved and often find that they have become full time carers by default. It is virtually impossible to measure and compare the human emotions and societal norms of duty, responsibility, love, guilt, commitment and so on, in a way that would provide us with some kind of index of the degree of free choice or compulsion involved in the process of becoming a carer. Many carers enjoy their work at least some of the time, and the majority are highly committed and emotionally attached to the person they care for. However, there are also differences in the prevalence of informal care work between socioeconomic groups, indicating that those with the option of purchasing care do often make use of that possibility either to supplement or to replace informal care inputs.

What kind of information do we have on the attitudes and beliefs of EU citizens regarding the question of who *should* be responsible for this care? The EU-wide survey referred to above also sought to establish what proportion of respondents would be willing to *increase* the responsibility of children for their parents care in old age. In the EU-15 as a whole, almost 60 percent of respondents were in favour of increased filial responsibility. However, the countries can be roughly divided into those that are very strongly in favour of increased family responsibility for aged parents and those that are less enthusiastic about such a prospect (Alber and Köhler 2004). Whereas in the Nordic countries, the Netherlands, Belgium and France less than half of the respondents were in favour of increasing adult children's responsibility, the percentage in favour of increased responsibility exceeded 60 percent in the Mediterranean countries and Ireland. The percentages in favour of increased responsibilities in individual countries varied from nearly 90 percent in Greece to approximately 30 percent in Sweden (Alber and Köhler 2004).

It is legitimate to assume that such differences in attitudes towards increased family responsibility reflect, to a large extent, not only cultural values but also the surrounding reality of service infrastructure. Where the alternatives to family care are extremely unappealing (expensive and/or low quality institutional care) it may be exceedingly distasteful and embarrassing to take recourse to them and very difficult to envisage significant improvements in such services. On the other hand, where formal services are well resourced, widely used and perceived to be of very high quality, the rationale for increasing family involvement may not be apparent, particularly where very high levels of labour market participation for both males and females make such increased family responsibility appear impractical.

As was pointed out above, the role of an informal carer is more frequently assumed by women than by men, and probably at a more demanding level (involving personal care) than the level usually assumed by men. Regarding the prospect of increased family responsibilities, can we detect a greater unwillingness among women to assume such responsibilities, as they would be more affected by such a change than men? The majority of women are against increasing family responsibility in only two EU countries, the Netherlands and Sweden. Across the EU as a whole, women are more likely than men to have a preference for increased family responsibility, a pattern that could be interpreted as altruism, adherence to traditional values, self-interest (fear of personally having to take recourse to low quality formal services), extreme distaste and distrust of formal services, or (most likely) a mixture of all these. Nonetheless, one can conclude from this, as Alber and Köhler do (2004: 71), that 'those who perform care work [in most countries] do not want to liberate themselves from this task and to externalise the cost of care to others, as a rational choice perspective might suggest'.

The future of informal care

It is frequently argued that developments such as declining family size, in other words, fewer adult children to look after ageing parents in combination with rising female labour market participation rates are making informal care increasingly scarce. Yet many countries (see below under the policy development case studies) continue to incentivize informal care. Does it make sense for policymakers to rely on continued supply of informal care services in the future? We will consider this question from both practical and normative viewpoints, in other words, we will answer the question of whether informal care is likely to be supplied in the future in quantities roughly similar to present levels, and whether relying on informal care is a good, or desirable, policy.

Employment status, presence of children and geographical distance from parents influence the likelihood of providing care to ageing parents (Wolf et al. 1997). To simplify somewhat, if an adult child is working, has children and especially if in addition to this he or she lives at a considerable distance from their ageing parent, their capacity to give (extensive, practical) care is clearly limited. Does the fact that labour market participation among women has increased, and many people move to obtain jobs mean that there is less scope for informal care giving, and that given the likely continuity of such trends, the scope for informal care giving is set to decrease for the foreseeable future?

All future developments are of course fundamentally unknowable. However, when attempting to predict future trends it makes sense to study past and present patterns and data pertaining to informal care, including care of other dependent population groups such as children. In childcare, the current pattern in many countries is somewhat bifurcated between parents who 'contract out' a large part of their childcare labour to formal childcare providers (thereby enabling themselves to work outside the home) and parents (largely mothers) who carry out the childcare work themselves, thereby precluding (full time) labour market participation. There is evidence that countries that support the working mother model have fared relatively well in terms of sustaining comparatively high fertility levels, which in turn suggests that women are most likely to reproduce in modern societies if they are given a genuine choice over whether, once mothers, they can work inside or outside the home (Castles 2003).

As Chapter 3 pointed out, the role of spouse carers is likely to increase and this group of carers is set to compensate to a large extent for the lesser availability of adult children in some cases to provide extensive care. In the case of 'adult child' carers, it appears likely that the future pattern will resemble the pattern in childcare – that there will be large numbers of those who will carry out this work themselves, but also large numbers of those who will 'contract out' the care of ageing parents (funded by the care recipient him/herself, by the adult children, or indeed jointly by both parties). In other words, for some segments of the population at least, there may be a shift from direct informal care giving to financial help with purchasing care (Johnson and Lo Sasso 2004). In those countries (especially the Nordic countries) where female labour market participation is already widespread and care services are either directly provided or financed to a large extent by the government, such 'contracting out' of heavy duty care is already widespread.

In answering the question 'should we rely on informal care?' from a normative perspective, a number of different considerations must be taken into account. It is clear that intensive care work limits other activities such as paid employment, hobbies and spending time with other family members and friends. Care work can also be physically dangerous: accidents can occur for instance when lifting the care recipient. Mental strain and extreme exhaustion can also result from looking after a person who may be prone to aggressiveness (a feature of some forms and stages of dementia) or require constant supervision, thereby leading to a lack of any spare time for the carer. Extreme role reversal and effective loss of the relationship can also occur in the case of dementia sufferers and their carers. Older carers in particular may be in a poor position to sustain the relentless and consuming nature of care work. As one person is typically responsible for the brunt of care work even in situations where other family members or formal respite care services allow for occasional breaks, care work can be very lonely and lead to social isolation. Exhaustion and isolation are particularly likely in situations where there is very limited support from formal service providers and where the care recipient (or the carer) is reluctant to accept outside help. In the light of these often very heavy costs that are internalized by informal carers, it can be argued that assigning all responsibility for care to a sole informal care giver is unethical in that it often has a detrimental impact on the carer's physical and mental health, and his or her opportunities for alternative activities including paid work and social engagement. The argument for ensuring that informal care is both voluntary and adequately supported by other (external) service is evident in the light of these considerations.

What are the policy implications of these concerns about the reliability and sustainability of future supplies of informal care? Policies should be more geared towards enabling people to combine, or alternate, between the roles of an informal carer and a worker. For those who wish to care on a permanent or full time basis, policies and benefits should enable sustained breaks from care work. Importance of (part time) work as a source of income and social contacts is great for carers who often end up on very low incomes and experience social isolation. In a small number of countries it is already possible to take some time off work or to adopt a more flexible working pattern when a close relative develops care needs. In countries where such entitlements are not available to everyone, some companies have developed arrangements for allowing employees to take time off or to work flexibly in cases where the employee wishes to devote time to the care of an older relative. Needless to say, such arrangements in the private sector tend to be available only to highly skilled employees whom the companies are keen to retain in the long run.

Who pays for care?

The financing of social care for older persons is no less complex than its provision: while the provider and financer are often indistinguishable (for instance, in the case of informal care the provider and de facto 'financer' is often a family member), these roles are increasingly bifurcated. There are many possible sources of financing the social care of older persons. Informal, family provided care can be financed by the family exclusively, or by some combination of the family absorbing some of the (opportunity) costs, and the government partially subsidizing the costs via for instance a carer's allowance or a cash for care benefit. For instance, in several countries (e.g., the Netherlands and Germany), cash for care and other types of long term care benefits can be channelled to a family carer or a formal provider (Timonen, Convery and Cahill 2006). With regard to formal care, the purchasers of this can be individuals or families or the government via a number of different universal or means tested payments, towards all, or part of the costs of care. These payments in turn can be tax or social insurance financed (Timonen 2005, 2006). Box 7.1 illustrates the different parties that can shoulder or share all or part of the costs of long term care for older people.

Box 7.1   The costs of long term care can be shouldered by, or shared between

- The *government* and/or *working population* (at the central or the local level, through taxes, social insurance or a combination of both).
- *Individuals* (through meeting the full cost from private income, savings and assets; by meeting part of the cost through co-payments and/or posthumous payments; or by taking out private insurance).
- *Families.*
- *Charities/voluntary organizations.*

Why is the division of responsibility for costs important?

In the mainstream healthcare services the protection of patients against 'catastrophic costs' is a widely accepted principle: in most developed countries, individuals (or their families) rarely pay the full or even any significant part of the cost of treating diseases such as cancer or heart disease 'out of their own pocket'. However, this is not the case with long term care. In many countries assets have to be run down to a considerable extent before public funding becomes available. The supply of care services in most countries (where it exists) free only for the worst off groups. While most Western welfare states combine public and private funding, there are great differences in the emphasis that they place on public versus private contributions towards the costs of care.

There are a number of reasons why the allocation of responsibility for meeting the costs of long term care is of great social and economic importance:

1   *Affordability* problems can lead to foregoing care even in the case of older people with extensive care needs: this is the most serious

problem associated with placing heavy emphasis on individual responsibility for financing the costs of care (Glendinning et al. 2004). While the problem of affordability is obviously most serious for low income individuals, the perception that care is 'too expensive' can also deter well off individuals from seeking care (in some cases due to pressure from family members to prevent the depletion of savings and assets that are expected as inheritance).

2 *Consistency*. The principle of protecting individuals and their families against 'catastrophic costs' (i.e., extremely high costs) in healthcare is well established and in most advanced industrialized countries people can receive treatment for most illnesses and diseases at no or very low cost. Why should the same principle not apply to long term care, or at least some elements of long term care?

3 *Efficiency*. The high cost of long term care in a system that offers healthcare at a considerably lower cost can lead to inappropriate care locations and use of resources. Covering healthcare costs but expecting individuals to bear the brunt of long term care costs can lead to excessive utilization of very expensive and excessively 'medicalized' healthcare as individuals seek to access affordable forms of care. A typical example of this is older people with relatively low care needs who seek hospital care due to the lack of any (affordable and accessible) alternatives in the community.

4 *Fairness*. If the risk of needing long term care is not pooled, some individuals and families are forced to shoulder extremely heavy costs. In systems that rely heavily on means testing or have vague eligibility rules that are inconsistently applied, some pay the bill themselves whereas others in broadly similar circumstances receive public assistance. While some individuals and families may be able to meet the costs of long term care without financial distress, the very high costs of long term care are a drain on the resources of most individuals and families.

5 *Long term planning*. It is extremely important that where long term care financing is not universally available (i.e., free or low cost to all who need care, regardless of their means), the rules governing eligibility for care and related benefits are clear and applied fairly and consistently. Such clarity enables long term planning by individuals and families, but is unfortunately lacking in many systems.

6 *Growing costs*. Population ageing in combination with the need to improve quality of long term care and remuneration levels for staff are likely to increase costs and to make the financing of long term care an increasingly acute policy issue.

The continuum of individual–family responsibility for the costs of care

In most developed countries there are some mechanisms in place for protecting individuals and families against the risk of having to meet the full costs of long term care. While in many countries individuals in residential (institutional) care have been exempted from meeting the costs of medical (nursing care), it is common practice to expect all or some individuals to meet all or part of the costs of their 'hotel costs' (accommodation and meals). However, at the time of writing, the author is not aware of any country where all long term care services would be completely free for those needing the services: Denmark comes closest as it offers home (domiciliary) care for free but charges accommodation costs in institutional care. The three most common practices are:

- *Universal entitlement with limited co-payments*: all individuals, regardless of their income, pay the same level of fees and other contributions. Alternatively, the fees may vary somewhat according to income, but there is a limit beyond which individuals are not responsible for the costs of their care. This is the practice in, for instance, Sweden and Finland.
- *Means testing to determine eligibility and co-payments that vary in accordance with income*: individuals above a means testing threshold are expected to finance their own care, those with means that fall below the threshold pay fees that are flat rate or vary in accordance with income. This is the practice, for instance, in England.
- *Defining the level of public support in accordance with non-monetary factors* such as care needs and dependency levels on the assumption that support from the government may not cover the costs of care fully. This is the practice in, for instance, Germany.

Note that under universal public programmes, the cost sharing is often quite substantial, but tends to be more evenly spread than in means tested programmes where those above the means testing limit shoulder all costs themselves. The long term care systems of the five countries that are discussed below represent all three basic models of individual responsibility for the costs of care (Timonen 2005).

Determinants of payment levels

A number of different factors can be taken into account in determining the level of individual contributions to the costs of care. The most commonly considered factors are:

- Income.
- Assets (savings, property).
- Degree of dependency (usually measured in terms of ability to carry out activities of daily living).
- Locus of care provision or the type of care provider (home/institution, formal/informal, public/private).
- Type of care/service (accommodation, nursing, personal care).

The two factors most commonly used in determining the costs of care or the contribution received from the government are income and the degree of dependency. The general trend in the OECD countries has in recent years been towards more extensive public contribution towards the costs of long term care. However, most countries are also attempting to contain the public long term care costs with the help of private cost sharing, targeting of benefits to those most in need, and strategies to delay the onset of disability in old age.

As was pointed out above, there are two main sources of financing public long term care expenditure:

- General taxation: most countries.
- Social insurance: Germany, Japan, Luxembourg, the Netherlands.

The OECD (2005) points out that a small number of countries provide relatively comprehensive coverage of the long term care needs of their populations in a way that could be seen as akin to the coverage of healthcare needs. Note that some of these countries operate social insurance funded and others operate tax funded programmes: it is clearly possible to achieve comprehensive coverage via both routes. Germany, Japan and Luxembourg have relatively recently adopted social insurance financed systems (the Netherlands has a longer standing insurance financed system), and Norway, Sweden and Austria have long term care programmes that are funded through general taxation.

In contrast to these seven countries with relatively comprehensive coverage, most countries currently have systems that depend in part or wholly on a means test of income and/or assets. In other words, entitlement to public care services and/or public support towards the costs of care depends on the ability of the individual to contribute towards the costs of their own care, with no or very little support being available to those who are assessed as having means above the income threshold. These countries include Canada, Hungary, Ireland, Korea, Mexico, New Zealand, Poland, Spain, Switzerland, the UK and the US. Public spending on long term care in these 'low coverage' countries varies between 0.2 and 1.5 percent of GDP, in contrast to the variance between 0.8 and 3 percent of GDP in the 'high coverage' countries (OECD 2005).

Germany, Japan, Sweden, the UK and the US represent all the main models of financing long term care and determining the eligibility for and the level of long term care cost sharing by individuals. Table 7.3 summarizes the funding arrangements and the extent of cost sharing by individuals in these countries.

Table 7.3 Long term care programmes, funding arrangements and cost sharing by individuals in Germany, Japan, Sweden, the UK and the US, 2005

Country	Name of programme	Funding	Cost sharing by individuals
Germany	Long term care insurance.	Insurance contributions.	Benefits are universal and non-means-tested; however, board and lodgings and other service charges in excess of a statutory limit are not covered; (where necessary these are covered by means tested social assistance).
Japan	Long term care insurance.	Insurance contributions and general taxation.	User co-payment 10% of total cost.
Sweden	Long term care services.	General taxation.	Moderate user fees set by local authorities within national maximum level.
UK	NHS and social services.	General taxation.	Users charged in accordance with ability to pay, but 'nursing care' free of charge for all.
US	Medicare and Medicaid.	Medicare: insurance contributions.	Medicare (nursing care only): first 20 days free, 20–100 days US$105 per day, 100% of cost after 100 days.
		Medicaid: general taxation.	Medicaid: low means testing threshold, co-payment charged according to ability to pay.

Table 7.4 sets out the main systemic features of long term care financing in our five case study countries. It is evident that these countries differ substantially in terms of the extent to which the responsibility for financing the costs of care is divided between individuals and the government, and the extent to which individuals are protected against 'catastrophic costs'.

Table 7.4 State/individual responsibility for the costs of long term care

Country	Government/individuals	Protection against catastrophic costs?
Sweden	Long standing emphasis on government responsibility for financing institutional care.	*Yes*. Clear maximum rates that can be charged and guaranteed amount that must be left over for personal expenses after care fees have been deducted.
Germany	Balance shifted from individuals towards the state, but individuals still expected to make heavy payments. Share financed by individuals is increasing as benefit rates have been kept constant since 1995 while the costs have increased substantially.	*Some* protection. Care insurance has eased the burden on many older people, but for charges over and above the amount covered by insurance they are still expected to run down income until social assistance threshold is reached.
US	Strong emphasis on individual responsibility.	*No*. Income and assets have to be depleted to a minimal level before any public assistance for care costs becomes available. Posthumous estate recovery possible.
UK	Strong emphasis on individual responsibility.	*Very limited* protection (assets up to £12,500 are protected).
Japan	Balance shifted towards the state.	*Yes*. Individuals responsible for paying 10% of the costs of care, and there is a maximum limit (dependent on income) that expenditure on user fees cannot exceed.

Care 'regimes'

While 'welfare regime classifications' (Esping-Andersen 1990) are widely accepted as reasonably valid and useful, and are extensively used in comparative welfare state analysis, 'systems' of care are difficult to classify into 'regimes' because the field of social care is inherently more complex and varied than that of cash benefits. Care services are rarely 'just' services, but can, and increasingly do, also involve a cash benefit element, for example, insurance or social assistance payments that cover the cost of care. It is also increasingly likely that the care service is delivered by someone other than the agency that finances it. As Anttonen, Sipilä and Baldock (2003) argue, social care is *universal but* there is great variety in forms and sources of care, ranging from 'direct' provision by public sector, to cash benefits with little regulation, to tax concessions, and so on.

Furthermore, regime classifications have tended to ignore some central features of care, such as the extensive reliance in many countries on informal care (see, for instance, Lewis 1992; Anttonen and Sipilä 1996; Esping-Andersen 1999). Esping-Andersen's regime classification was criticized for gender blindness, and for concentrating on the income protection of wage earners in formal employment relationships (Hobson 1990; Lewis 1992; Orloff 1993; Sainsbury 1994). As Daly (2001: 37) points out 'even in the most advanced welfare states, caring is never completely provided in the formal (professional) settings'. A good starting point in constructing social care regimes is an acknowledgement that remarkably little is known about even the most basic aspects of informal care, such as the quantity of care and who provides the care. Even the formal care services sector tends to be a complex field of research, as these services are often organised in a decentralized way and statistics are rarely aggregated at the national level in a reliable and helpful way. In many countries data on care provision and expenditure has to be collated from a disparate range of sources, often at different (federal, regional, state, local, etc.) levels of government (whereas data on income transfers tend to be available from a single, centralized source). These problems are inevitably magnified when trying to compile data from a wide range of countries, although some progress has recently been made in this regard (see OECD 2005).

Following the recognition that the three worlds of welfare capitalism are not entirely satisfactory for the purposes of classifying (and understanding) social care systems, a number of valuable attempts have been made to develop systematic ways of thinking about social care. Steps towards identifying services as a separate area of policy analysis were initially taken by Kohl (1981). Kohl's analysis of social expenditure and investment in services vis-à-vis cash benefits or transfers led him to highlight the dichotomy between *service* states and *transfer* states. The former tend to be coterminous with the Scandinavian countries, and the latter with continental-corporatist welfare states (see also Kautto 2002).

Alber (1995) recommends that the supply of social services to older people be analysed and compared using three variables: first, expenditure on such services; second, the number of residential and domiciliary care services;

and, third, the take-up rate of these services. However, the difficulty involved in obtaining accurate national representative statistics in relation to these areas tends to restrict analysis to countries that are more advanced in the collection of such statistics. Furthermore, while this information is useful, it does not elucidate the reasons for the variation between different social care systems. To explain this variation, Alber recommends further analysis of care systems under four broad headings. These are the regulatory structure, the financial structure, the structure of supply, and the degree of consumer power.

In their work, Anttonen and Sipilä (1996: 87) set out to 'bring social care services into the domain of comparative social policy research' arguing that 'comparative research into social care services has not, as yet, made very impressive progress'. Drawing on small scale empirical analysis of care services for children and older people, and on data on women's labour market participation rates, Anttonen and Sipilä (1996) identified two distinct models of social care services: the Scandinavian model of public services and the (Mediterranean) family care model. Two other, more tentative, models were also identified. These were the British means tested model and the Central European subsidiarity model.

Drawing on these classifications and on data relating to developments in the 1990s in France, Spain, England, Sweden and Germany, Timonen (2005) identified three broad paradigms in the area of long term care services for older people. The first of these is the 'statist' paradigm, where the government takes extensive responsibility for financing and providing long term care. The second is the 'familial/individualist' paradigm of long term care, where families and individuals are responsible for financing long term care and where services available through the state are means tested and limited to a small proportion of the older population. In the third, referred to as 'state pays, others provide' paradigm of long term care, the government funds all or part of the costs of care while multiple players engage in the delivery of services (family, voluntary and private sector). In other words, there is a clear 'purchaser–provider' division. The parallels between these paradigms and two of the four models identified by Anttonen and Sipilä (1996) are clear; the family care and means tested models are here collapsed into one (the familial/individualist model).

Box 7.2 Social care regimes/models

- *Scandinavian model of public services*: services for older people widely available; women's labour market participation very high; independence of local governments as can levy taxes; universalism.
- *Family care model*: Portugal, Spain, Greece and Italy: most services produced

on informal or grey market; the better off use private services; public authorities play a modest role.

Possibly also:

- *British means tested model*: moving towards residuality. (Ireland between the Southern European and British model.)
- *Central European subsidiarity model* in the case of old age welfare: Netherlands and Germany (Belgium and France): family has primary responsibility; role of voluntary organizations; health insurance a major source of funding.

Source: Anttonen and Sipilä (1996).

Developments in long term care policy

While regime classifications are helpful in simplifying the complexity of social care of older people they are of limited value in trying to capture the recent dynamics of change in this policy area (Doyle and Timonen 2007). Anttonen, Baldock and Sipilä (2003: 171) acknowledge that 'to suggest that nations are even preponderantly of one mode of provision or another ... is to underestimate diversity in each country'. Long term care policy is at present one of the most frequently changing policy areas and as such it is possible to give only a snapshot of recent developments in a small number of countries.

Germany

Germany introduced a long term care insurance scheme in 1994. The decision to establish this new social insurance scheme was arguably motivated first and foremost by the increased cost of social assistance for frail older persons. Financing social assistance is the responsibility of the *Länder* in Germany, and their increasing unwillingness to finance long term care, combined with the popularity of a new care insurance scheme among the electorate, constituted powerful incentives to construct a federal scheme.

The German long term care insurance benefits are not indexed, and were not designed to cover all costs of long term care – some elements of cost control were therefore built into the design of the system from the start. In order to try to prevent shift from informal (family) and home-based to formal and institutional care, a range of options were offered to support home care, including a cash payment for the informal carer.

The German long term insurance system has arguably reduced the dependency of frail older persons on their relatives (Aust and Bönker 2004), and as such represents a shift of responsibility (if not necessarily agency) from the sphere of family to the state. The long term care insurance is financed through social insurance contributions amounting to a maximum of 1.7 percent of gross income (shared equally between the employer and the employee). There is a growing gap between payments (fixed since 1995) and cost of care. Inadequacies of the long term care insurance, in combination with financial pressures, are generating a situation where a major reform of the system appears likely.

France

Like most other countries, France did not have a benefit system specifically directed at older people in need of long term care until the late 1990s. Reports in the late 1980s and early 1990s made the case for a benefit scheme specifically designed for older people, and a wide political consensus developed on the need for such a benefit (Mandin and Palier 2003). The *prestation spécifique dependence* (PSD) was created in 1997. This benefit was targeted to people 60 years of age or older, and the amount was dependent both on financial means and the degree of dependence.

However, the PSD soon came under heavy criticism. A report published in May 2000 criticized the low take-up rates of the benefit (due to the means testing process, loss of assets and lack of information), the inadequate level of services provided by pension insurance funds, and the great variation in the rules and conditions between different local authority areas (Mandin and Palier 2003). The PSD was also criticized for not covering the actual costs of long term care. As in other countries, the drawing of lines between private and public responsibilities proved to be the most controversial aspect of reforming the long term care benefit in France. The take-up of the PSD was low because older persons in need of the benefit preferred to forego it rather than see their assets (i.e., their children's inheritance) being diminished or completely depleted. Following a reform the long term care benefit and the creation of the *allocation personnalisée d'autonomie* (APA) in 2002, assets were excluded from the means test and the creation of a new insurance scheme was rejected on grounds of cost.

The degree of autonomy in activities of daily living and income of the applicant determine the level of APA payable. The benefit is paid either in cash or in the form of subvention to an institution, or as vouchers to the carer (*titres emplois-services*). The exclusion of assets from the means test has meant that APA is an expensive scheme, and its cost have indeed been the main reason for criticism of the APA. Regional councils threatened increases in local taxes on the grounds that the scheme was not adequately financed. Some cutback measures were introduced in 2003, reflecting the difficulty of introducing an adequate new benefit under the conditions of 'permanent austerity', even when such a benefit is a response to a widely acknowledged social need (Mandin and Palier 2003).

Spain

Informal family care is the predominant mode of care provision for older people in Spain. There has been no decisive policy innovation or experimentation at the central level, but the regional governments (*Comunidades Autónomas*) have introduced some schemes for health and social care of older people (Moreno 2004). As a result, there are 17 different regional systems for helping older people to meet their long term care needs, each with different operating principles, objectives and funding mechanisms. Some tax relief has also been introduced for carer households, and this seems a more likely direction of future reform than direct spending. In areas where women are no longer able or willing to provide care services free of charge, private companies and (to a lesser extent) non-profit organizations are projected to assume a greater role (Moreno 2004). The residential care sector is already dominated by the private sector (with 70 percent of places being run by private companies), and the role of the private sector is increasing in the home help and day centre sectors.

England

Long term care services are financed through general taxation and out of pocket payments in the UK. Virtually all nursing and residential care homes are private (for profit and not for profit), and subject to a charge depending on income *and* assets.

The Royal Commission on Long-Term Care argued in its findings published in 1999 that risk pooling was required in the area of long term care, but rejected both public and private insurance, recommending instead that nursing *and* personal care costs be covered by general taxation (Royal Commission 1999). The Commission argued that as the NHS covered the nursing costs of those in hospital care due to illness or disease, it would be illogical and unfair to charge people in long term care for the costs of similar care. The UK government accepted that the NHS should cover the nursing costs of people in long term care, but rejected the argument that 'personal' care should be covered. The government did, however, agree to modify the means testing with a view to reducing its impact in 2001/02.

The cost of nursing home care in the UK is very high. According to the new means testing rules, those with assets (including savings, investments and property[2]) worth more than €30,000 (£20,000) are not eligible for state support. Those with assets worth £12,250–£19,999 pay a share that varies with income. Those with assets worth less than £12,250 receive state funding. Consequently, individuals with savings and assets are expected to spend these down to the social assistance means test level before receiving any public subsidy.

The purchaser–provider distinction is well established in the UK: nursing homes and local governments negotiate rates for public patients. However, some providers seek to recoup income by charging more from private patients. The recent decline in the size of the private institutional care sector has been attributed by some to insufficient payments for the care of public patients. The UK government's response to the care home closures, namely the substantial increases in funding channelled to the care homes in combination with the retreat on the National Care Standards, is a warning example to other countries where service provision is highly dependent on the cooperation of private sector companies (see Netten et al. 2005). The success of the National Service Framework for Older People in bringing about more 'person centred' care is yet to be properly assessed (Department of Health (UK) 2001).

Japan

The long term care insurance scheme that was introduced in Japan in 2000 covers all residents aged 40 or over, for both home-based and institutional care. One of the main aims of the new scheme was to reduce inappropriate hospitalization and rising health insurance costs that resulted from the 'social hospitalization' of older people who entered hospital care when no informal care was available (Hiraoka 2004).[3] The new insurance scheme represented a radical break from the traditional care model in Japan that was largely based on informal family care, and made Japan the first Asian country where the state has substantial responsibility for meeting the costs of long term care. The Japanese long term care reform is the most radical reform that has been implemented by any country in this policy area, and serves as a proof of the feasibility of extensive, system transforming policy changes.

Fifty percent of the cost of long term care insurance in Japan is covered by general taxation, 32 percent by employee contributions, and 18 percent by pensioner contributions. There is no single rate of contribution: municipalities levy contributions that are needed to cover the costs. Employee and pensioner contributions are graduated by income (with a maximum limit), and social assistance funds subsidize the contributions of those on low incomes.

The service user pays 10 percent of the cost of services and the remainder of costs is borne by municipalities. Benefits are received as an equivalent amount of services. Approximately three-quarters of recipients opt for home care, and one-quarter choose institutional care. The scheme has yielded some positive results such as enhancing the choice of services and increasing in-home care services: the number of service users has increased substantially since the introduction of the scheme in 2000.

It has been estimated that average contributions to the Japanese long term care insurance may have to increase by 80 percent over the next ten years (OECD 2005). Prevention ('healthy ageing') strategies are being urgently developed in order to reduce demand for long term care.

United States

In the United States, those who can afford it are expected to meet their own long term care costs (except acute care nursing which is covered by Medicare). Medicaid, a means tested social assistance programme (funded through general taxation) pays the costs of those who cannot afford to pay themselves. Recent policies have encouraged more extensive use of Medicaid for paying for home and community care services with the aim of preventing entry into (more expensive) nursing home care. While the private long term care insurance market is expanding, it still covers only 15 percent of the 65+ population with incomes of US$20,000 or higher. Approximately 94 percent of nursing homes in the United States are private, and two-thirds of these are for profit (Scharlach 2007).

Sweden

Long term care services in Sweden are tax financed and universally available to all who are assessed as being in need of care. User charges apply, however, and these were raised in the 1990s but capped in 2002. 'Maximum charges' (*maxtaxa*) now apply to both home care and institutional care, and within this upper limit the costs to individuals vary in accordance with the type of care, the number of hours of care received, the standard of accommodation (in the case of institutional care) and taxable income.

A reform undertaken in 1992 made municipalities (local authorities) responsible for the cost of delayed discharges from hospitals: municipalities are now expected to find community or residential care for older people being discharged from hospital, and to foot the bill of continued hospital care where no such long term care can be arranged. Whereas in 1990 approximately 15 percent of hospital beds were occupied by 'delayed discharges', in 1999 this percentage had fallen to 6 percent. Due to the pressure to contain expenditure, the trend in Sweden over the last ten years has been towards targeting services for sicker and more disabled older people than in the past: as a result, more medicalized care is provided for fewer people. However, the proportions of older people receiving both home care and institutional care are still very high in international comparison (OECD 2005).

Since 2002, older people in need of long term care have been protected against high user fees. Before the reform municipalities were charging different amounts, some considerably more than others. Maximum fees for home care, day centres, healthcare and different forms of residential care are now clearly defined, as is the amount of 'spending money' that must be left over for personal purchases after the fees, accommodation costs and taxes have been paid (Socialstyrelsen 2003). The user fees vary according to income, but a national maximum level caps them effectively. If the amount left over is smaller than the legally required minimum, user charges are reduced accordingly. The 'spending money' is intended to cover costs such as telephone bills, hairdressing, chiropody, newspapers and magazines, clothes, presents, medicines and travel. Note that property and assets are not taken into account: the system is designed to benefit, and to gain the approval of, all income groups.

Increasing employment rates and thereby generating more revenue is the preferred option as there is great reluctance to lower the level of service provision: note that high employment levels among women contribute towards a broad tax base but also necessitate extensive care services provision for children and dependent adults. There is great concern to make the public care services sector a more attractive employer as staff shortages are severe in some parts of the country, particularly in sparsely populated areas (Timonen 2005).

Conclusion

Social care services for older people are a highly complex and fascinating area of study. Long term care in many countries is an intricate mosaic of public and private responsibilities for the provision and financing of care. Indeed, social care has been called 'a barometer of the balance of the public and private worlds within a society' (Sipilä et al. 2003: 2). This chapter has outlined the basic concepts that are used in making sense of this complex balance, and has sought to illustrate the fact that while care is clearly ubiquitous, it is also extremely diverse. Furthermore, long term care is a constantly evolving policy area, with many countries in recent times having transformed their care systems as a result of various social, political and economic pressures (Fine 2007). Comprehensive systems (whether tax or insurance based) for financing long term care of older people have proved extremely popular wherever they have been introduced, notwithstanding various challenges in ensuring their sustainability and adequacy. Private insurance on its own does not seem to be a reliable alternative, but can act as a useful addition to public insurance (it has proven quite popular in Germany for instance). While long term care is still widely perceived as costly, many politicians and policy-makers have come to appreciate the cost savings in other areas, especially in healthcare, that can be achieved with the help of well designed 'social' care systems that prevent and delay entry into highly expensive residential and hospital care. We will now turn, in Chapter 8, to discussing the home, community and institutional care settings, and the relative emphasis that different countries have placed on these.

Notes

1   Note that this figure includes care provided to relatives and outside the kinship system, and all categories of adult care recipients such as older people and people with a disability or a long term illness.
2   Except when the individual's spouse or partner continues to live in the house. There is also a three-month property disregard: for the first three months after admission into residential care, the value of the patient's home is disregarded in the means test. Funds have been made available to local councils to provide loans to older people who need care but are not willing to sell their homes.
3   Note the parallel here to the rationale for introducing the German long term care insurance: reducing the cost of other programmes, especially in the social assistance system.

8 Care services for older people II: community and institutional care

Introduction

'Institutional' and 'community' care are frequently employed terms that are nonetheless poorly understood. Chapter 7 has already indicated that only a small proportion of older people need and receive institutional care, and that the majority of those in need of care receive it in their own homes or in 'the community', in most countries predominantly from family members but also (and increasingly) from formal (paid) service providers. The previous chapter also elaborated at length on the informal–formal distinction and the contributions of informal (family) carers: this chapter focuses on *formal* care services only. As increasing numbers of older people are likely to receive formal care in the future (either in parallel with or instead of informal care), it is of great importance to understand where and how this care is provided. Quality controls and service user participation in decisions about care are inadequate or lacking in many countries, and constitute areas that require urgent attention by policymakers and practitioners. The lack or inadequacy of quality controls in care services for older people that is evident in many countries reflects the attitude that different, less exacting standards apply to older people than to children for example.

The locations of formal care

Formal care, in other words, care provided by paid carers who are not related to the care recipient, can take place in the older person's home (domiciliary care), in the 'community' surrounding that home or in a separate location that is usually an institution ('nursing home' or other residential setting). In practice, the distinctions between these different loci are blurred, at least in some countries. For instance, countries as different in their social and care policies as Denmark and the United States both have highly developed assisted and supported living sectors: it is difficult to know whether these should be classified as home (or home-like) care settings, as institutional settings, or as something in between. In Denmark these settings are mostly owned by the (local) government while in the United States there exists a large market for privately purchasing or renting 'retirement homes' in communities that often offer a 'continuum of care' from light-touch housekeeping services to full nursing care. While the homes in these communities therefore often closely resemble 'normal' homes, they can incorporate a range of housing options from fully independent housing to a nursing care facility.

Due to the great diversity of care settings, the involvement of multiple state level, regional, county and municipal actors in the provision and financing of services, and the lack of systematic data collection on service provision at the national level, researching and collecting data on formal care (and especially home and community care) is extremely challenging in most countries. These challenges are compounded when conducting cross-country comparative research on care (Scharf and Wenger 1995). However, in recent years some comparative data on the financing and provision of formal care services has become available – we will now turn to examining this.

Publicly provided and financed formal care

Two commonly used indicators of the extent of service provision by care providers other than informal carers are the percentage of older people receiving home help services and the percentage of older people in institutional care. While these are useful indicators, they also have limitations. The proportion of the older (65+) population in receipt of formal home care services and institutional care varies considerably between countries, as can be seen from Table 8.1. Note, however, that these figures (as is the case for most comparative datasets relating to long term care) only relate to care services that are *publicly* provided or financed from the public purse. An individual who receives home help or is resident in an institution may be paying for some or all of that care themselves (or their family may be held financially responsible). These figures also exclude home care provision by informal (family) carers. Around one-fifth of Norwegian and British older people are in receipt of government funded domiciliary care, in contrast to under 3 percent of older people in the United States. While this does mean that a much smaller proportion of people are in receipt of formal care services sponsored or provided by the government, it does not necessarily mean that the *overall* proportion of older persons in receipt of some form of care in their own home is considerably lower. The lower coverage of formal services is doubtlessly compensated by informal (family) care, although in the absence of comprehensive data we cannot be sure of the precise extent of this compensation.

Table 8.1 also shows that differences between countries tend to be greater in the area of community care provision: whereas the percentage of older

Table 8.1. Percentage of 65+ receiving institutional and home care services, selected countries, most recent year for which data is available (c. 2000)

Country	% of 65+ in receipt of home help	% of 65+ in institutional care
Australia	14.7	5.3
Austria	14.8	3.6
Germany	7.1	3.9
Ireland	c. 5	4.6
Japan	5.5	3.2
Netherlands	12.3	2.4
Norway	18.0	6.0
Sweden	9.1	7.9
UK	20.3	5.1
US	2.8	4.3

Source: OECD (2005).

people in institutional care does not vary dramatically between countries, the differences in the proportion receiving formal (public or state funded) home care are remarkable (see also Jacobzone 2000). The OECD (2005) estimates that publicly provided or financed home help is almost non-existent (with only around 1 percent of the older population receiving home help) in Greece, Italy, New Zealand, Portugal and Spain. Countries with modest levels of formal home help include the United States, Germany, Ireland and Japan (although in the United States coverage varies between the States from 0 to approximately 8 percent). Significant levels of home help provision can be found in Australia, Austria, Belgium, France and the Netherlands. High levels of provision in terms of coverage of the older population are found in the United Kingdom and the Nordic countries. Note, however, that similarities in *coverage* can mask great differences in the *level* of service provision: the amount of services that the average older home care user in, say, Denmark, receives, is far higher than the amount of services devoted to an average recipient in the United Kingdom. It is much harder, however, to achieve such detailed comparability in cross-country statistics, for the reasons pointed out above.

Data compiled by the OECD (2005) show that there is a weak link between the proportion of the older population in institutional care and the proportion of older persons receiving some form of (publicly funded) home care. Roughly speaking, as the proportion of the older population in institutional care increases, so does the proportion who are receiving home care services. In other words, countries that offer a lot of institutional care also tend to offer domiciliary services to a comparatively large proportion of their older population. Most of the countries with lowest levels of home care also have particularly low levels of institutional care. There is therefore no pattern of substitution between institutional and home care. In a handful of countries, the balance of service provision could be said to be clearly in favour of home care (Denmark, Australia, Austria, Norway and the UK).

There is a clear tendency for the use of home care services to increase with age, but also considerable variation between countries in this respect. Increasingly, services are more heavily concentrated on the oldest old (i.e., people who require both personal care and assistance in managing the household).

We will first briefly discuss some of the key issues associated with institutional care before turning to a more detailed discussion of home and community care.

Institutional care

While institutional care arguably has some inherent difficulties that are hard to address, there is no reason in principle why residential care cannot be of high quality and designed in a person centred way that enhances the residents' quality of life (Peace et al. 1997). Unfortunately, however, institutional care has tended to suffer from many problems. Many institutional care settings operate on the basis of the assumption that older people have uniform needs. Residents are often treated as passive recipients of care, and priority is placed in physical care and routine tasks such as feeding, bathing, making the bed and distributing medications (timing of which is dictated by staff rotas rather than the residents' preferences). Institutional care tends to revolve around a set routine for all residents; many institutions lack single rooms (or double rooms for couples) or indeed any privacy; care plans are frequently not individualized; and there can be a reluctance to refer residents for diagnosis or assessment of medical conditions. As a result, emphasis is often on treatment of symptoms (sometimes involving overly heavy use of psychotropic medications) rather than on rehabilitation. It is frequently assumed that older people only have physical and health needs, and either no or only very modest social and 'higher level' needs (such as the need to influence their surroundings and have a say in decisions concerning them). This is reflected in the lack of or insufficient availability of psychological and social work services. Little attention is often paid to social activity, education or creative activities and where they exist, they can be highly unimaginative and overly structured (prayers on Sundays, bingo on Tuesdays and so on). Older people are sometimes 'infantilized' in residential care by (well-meaning) staff who call them by their first name or by 'pet' names ('dear'). Rarely are residents in institutional care allowed to make decisions about their own care and there can be an overemphasis on protection and safety. Conflicting priorities can easily arise in institutional care: cleanliness, order and 'safety' typically override independence and activities that are seen as involving risk taking (such as outings to the outside world).

Many countries have no national standards of residential care, and sometimes not even voluntary codes of practice. Happily, in others reasonable progress has been made in ensuring good quality institutional care. For instance, the UK Care Standards Act (Department of Health (UK) 2001) establishes minimum standards and independent inspections of all private and voluntary nursing homes and residential institutions, sets targets for the proportion of carers who should be qualified and provides detailed core requirements which apply to all care homes. 'Whistle blowing' protection for staff who alert authorities to the failures of the system is vital if care workers are to be encouraged to speak out without fear of putting their jobs at risk: such protections have been introduced in Sweden for instance.

Home and community care: like motherhood and apple pie?

Despite the potential to provide good quality residential care, nursing homes and similar institutional care settings are almost universally unpopular. The popularity of home care is evident from the fact that in the EU (both EU-15 and EU-25) over 80 percent of people prefer domiciliary care services (Alber and Köhler 2004). As Chapter 7 pointed out, the allocation of preferences for formal or informal providers in the home care setting varies considerably between countries. The availability and quality of care exert a strong influence on these attitudes: formal services tend to be considerably more popular and accepted in countries that have invested in developing this sector in a way that ensures quality services to a significant proportion of the older population in need of care. When services are used by a large number of people who are by and large satisfied with them, the popularity of services tends to increase. Means tested services in combination with poor systems of quality assurance and monitoring tend to make formal care highly unpopular and even feared especially by older people who (often rightly) have concerns about the quality of care provided by formal sector carers.

The shift in emphasis from institutional care to care in the community and in the home has been slow to evolve but is now commonly and firmly promoted by policymakers and advocates of 'ageing in place', or 'maintien à domicile', including older persons who, for the most part, have a preference for home care. In the light of population ageing, changes in family structures, an increase in women's labour market participation rates and the perceived unsuitability and high cost of institutional care, the challenge of providing adequate community care has become a policy concern of great importance.

Chapter 4 pointed out that while the *proportion* of people in the older age groups in need of care appears to be declining, at least in some countries and some population groups (see Fries 2003 for instance), the *absolute number* of older people requiring care will increase in the short and medium term. Most countries have made the decision at least in principle that, whenever possible, such care should take place in the older person's home. While it is certainly ill-advised to make very pessimistic predictions about the availability of help and care from informal sources, there can be little doubt that the demand for *formal* home care services is set to increase significantly. In this context, it is important to understand the ways in which home care is organized, financed and delivered to older people in different policy contexts.

The policy aspiration of virtually all countries is therefore to ensure that the majority of older people can stay in their own homes and communities for as long as possible, even when care needs arise. While it is possible to take a cynical stance on this and argue that such aspirations have remained largely unfulfilled and are driven primarily by cost considerations (the often mis-guided belief that home care, whether formal or informal, is 'cheap'), it is nonetheless, broadly speaking, positive that such aspirations exist and have in some cases been fulfilled. Indeed, it has been shown that home adaptations and assistive technologies installed in the home, not only can close the gap between functional ability and suitability of the home environment, but can also result in economies arising from the reduced need for formal care services (although the length of use of the adapted home and the presence or absence of an informal carer naturally influence the results of the cost–benefit cal-culation in individual cases) (Lansley et al. 2004). In addition to cost con-siderations, the promotion of home care is rooted in consideration of the quality of life of older persons. It is important to note that preference for care in the home does not always equal preference for care by family members – it appears that care by formal care givers is increasingly acceptable to older people who are not as averse to formal services as is frequently argued. Also, very different alternatives to care in the older person's own home (such as moving to a relative's home and institutional setting) can be equally unpa-latable for older people (Garavan et al. 2001).

There are several dangers, however, in the almost universal exhortation to shift to home and community care. First, home and community care is easily equated with informal (family) care with the attendant result that it is de facto ignored by policymakers (see Chapter 7 for a discussion of problems associated with unsupported family care). Second, and related to the first point, home and community care is often (wrongly) seen as a 'cheap' policy direction leading to underinvestment in the sector. Third, it is sometimes assumed (again wrongly) that home and community care are both impossible to regulate and do not need as much regulation and quality control as institutional care (Ahern et al. 2007). As Qureshi and Walker (1998) have pointed out, it is likely that both the best and worst examples of care can be found in the domestic sphere, and it is therefore important to ensure that quality of domiciliary care is monitored as rigorously as the quality of institutional care.

When these reservations are combined, at worst the simplistic exhortation to provide home and community care can result in very poor levels of service provision and inadequate support for informal carers, lack of quality controls and ultimately (unintentionally) diverting people to institutional care as a result of the shortcomings in home and community care. In other words, advocacy of home and community care can become akin to advocating motherhood and apple pie – well meaning but vacuous.

Home and community care

What then is this 'home and community care' that has become so popular and is almost universally seen to be worth striving for? The umbrella term 'home and community care' comprises a wide variety of services that are delivered in the older person's home or in a communal setting. Typical *home*, or *domiciliary*, care services are personal care (assistance with washing, dressing, toileting, taking meals and other tasks pertaining to the maintenance of normal daily activities of living) and assistance with domestic work such as cleaning and cooking (these will be elaborated on below). Typical *community* care services are 'daycare centres' that can offer a mix of social activities, meals and other services such as hairdressing or chiropody. While more 'medical' in orientation, community (or public health) nursing and general practitioner (family doctor) services form important components of 'care in the community'. A range of other professionals, such as physiotherapists and occupational therapists can also be involved in maintaining an older person in their own home, typically through short term rehabilitation following a hospital stay or period of illness, or during a period of adapting the home for the older person's changed needs (for instance by identifying the home adaptations and assistive devices that an older person requires in order to continue living at home and training them to use such equipment).

Home and community care services are underdeveloped in many countries. This is arguably a legacy of the fact that, until relatively recently, home and community care was in most countries exclusively provided by families and other informal actors: due to its highly private and 'hidden' nature, this care has traditionally not been the focus of public policies (Fine 2007). The services that tend to be particularly underdeveloped include specialized social work services for older people, speech and language therapy, nutrition advice and chiropody. The lack of (both community- and hospital-based) social workers is highly problematic, as social workers would be well placed to act as the key professionals who could refer older people to other service providers such as home helps, public health nurses, meals on wheels, respite care, day centres and voluntary sector agencies that in many countries act as important service providers.

It is obvious from the description above that home and community care comprises a very wide variety of services and a wide array of professionals, both medical and social care, delivering those services. It should also be pointed out that informal (family) and formal carers are increasingly providing care in tandem, not least as a result of programmes that enable the care recipient to use their entitlements to 'cash for care' and similar payments to 'hire' both family members and formal carers (Ungerson 2004; Glendinning 2006). It would be impossible to discuss the full range and variety of home and community care in one chapter. As the purpose of this book is to provide an introduction to some of the most relevant and topical areas of policy, we will here focus on formal home, or domiciliary, care.

Home (domiciliary) care

Formal domiciliary (home) care services are a good example of policies and services adapting to population ageing; when they were first introduced, they were typically designed to alleviate the workload and stress of mothers with newborn children and/or large families. In recent decades, their focus has in many countries shifted away from families with young children and towards older people (Doyle and Timonen 2007).

Cullen et al. (2004) offer a useful typology that helps to define the parameters of domiciliary or home care. According to their typology, care can be broken down into four categories:

- *Practical*: for example, domestic tasks such as preparing a meal, cleaning the house and doing shopping.
- *Personal*: for example, washing and bathing, help with getting dressed and providing continence care.
- *Monitoring/supervision*: for example, of persons with dementia who may be confused when using appliances or in danger of wandering.
- *Care management*: providing support through management activities such as liaising with health professionals and coordinating care services.

It is evident, therefore, that home care, and care work in the home, are extremely diverse. Persons who require domiciliary care services usually have a limitation in 'activities of daily living' (ADL) such as washing, dressing or eating, and/or in 'instrumental activities of daily living' (IADL) such as shopping, cleaning or meal preparation. Home carers often deliver many different types of care, comprising assistance with ADL and IADL but also allied tasks such as prompting medication, and often equally important social functions such as keeping company and discussing any worries or concerns of the older person. Whether or not an older person with ADL/IADL difficulties is eligible for state funded domiciliary care services varies according to the regulations in a specific country: in some instances, eligibility is determined on the basis of income and assets, in others, the degree of ADL limitations determines eligibility, and in other systems a combination of both means and functional ability is used to determine eligibility.

Formal home care can be provided by many different types of care workers. Home care services are provided in some countries by public sector employees working for a municipality or a similar unit of local government, but increasingly local governments are contracting services out to (for profit and not for profit) providers who have to compete for these contracts. In practice categories such as *medical* and *non-medical* or *social* care workers are often blurred. In the United States for instance, home carers in California's largest home care programme, the In-Home Supportive Services, can perform paramedical tasks such as dispensing medication, dressing wounds and administering injections; in Germany informal carers who are paid through the long term care insurance programme can deliver paramedical services (once trained to do so); but in Denmark paramedical care services are the preserve of qualified nurses (Doyle and Timonen 2007). In many countries, migrant care workers operating outside the formal economy have come to play an increasingly important role in providing home care to older people. Given the recency of this development, very little is known of this kind of care work, which may become very widespread as a result of the joint forces of international migration, service (or funding) shortages and population ageing.

Terminology surrounding home care also varies across and within different countries. For example, Tester (1996: 5) points out that 'the concept of "community care" also [and perhaps especially] comprises home care in the UK, and home care is commonly referred to as "community-based long-term care" in the US'. Also, in the United States home carers can be called 'home makers', 'care givers' or 'providers'. In Ireland they are called 'home helps' or personal care assistants or attendants (Timonen, Doyle and Prendergast 2006). In the UK and Australia they are called 'carers', while in India and some other countries they are called 'care takers' (WHO 2002). Similarly, whereas home care recipients are typically referred to as consumers in the United States, in other (Anglophone) countries they are referred to as home care beneficiaries, service users or care recipients.

Policy developments

While long term care policies vary greatly between countries, there are certain general trends that are shared by several countries with relatively developed formal care systems. In several countries, it has been decided that competition and enterprise should be stimulated in the area of long term care provision. It is possible to argue that such attempts are rooted in employment policy, particularly in countries that have determined to create (predominantly low wage, part time) jobs in the service sector (Morel 2006). It is also argued that competition between providers would serve the purpose of offering choice and flexibility to service users. For a range of reasons, countries such as the Netherlands (personal budgets), England (direct payments), and Italy have adopted systems that strive to achieve the multiple aims of giving service users 'consumer power', fostering new businesses and generating employment, and possibly even helping to control public expenditure. These programmes are sometimes given the collective label of 'cash for care' (Ungerson 2004), denoting policies that channel funds ('cash') to persons in need of care, who then exercise varying degrees of choice in selecting providers to whom these payments are given in exchange for care provision. Cash for care policies (alongside 'standard' programmes such as the long term care insurance in Germany) have been criticized for inadequacy of payments, insufficient quality controls and limited extent of choice. These possible weaknesses notwithstanding, cash for care arrangements are interesting for the changes in thinking in care policy that they represent, and they are likely to be extended as social markets and the principle of consumer control gain ground (Timonen et al. 2006).

In many countries, the focus is still on providing medical care rather than long term care. This is based on the assumption that the public sector's proper remit is in the provision of medical care, and other types of care can more appropriately (and 'cheaply') be provided by unpaid family members and the voluntary sector. An unintended result of such thinking is often the overutilization of expensive forms of (hospital and other institutional) care and extreme forms of carer stress (see Chapter 7). Even where formal care services are available, there is often an 'in-built' bias towards institutional care that is created by the structure of entitlements and benefits. For instance, older people may be entitled to apply for funding to finance nursing home care, but there is no similar entitlement to help with paying for home and community care services. In practice, older people with extensive needs often have to choose between staying at home, with little or no public support, and full time residential (nursing home) care. Ideally, of course, there should be a range of options for older people and their families.

Where formal home and community care services are developed, they are often insufficiently focused on fostering independence. For instance, an older person with some mobility difficulties may be offered a 'home help' who does the shopping instead of being offered physiotherapy and transport and assistive devices that would enable him or her to continue to do his or her own shopping. A better mix of preventive, acute, rehabilitation and long term care services for older people is therefore needed.

In Denmark, often held up as the model country for home and community care provision, new institutional care settings can only be built in exceptional cases. The favoured concept is 'elder friendly housing' coupled with services delivered to the place of residence. Home care does not merely entail older people remaining in their original homes. Home care is available, where needed, throughout the day.

In the UK, the Community Care Act of 1990 (implemented from April 1993) was prompted by a concern over the dramatic rise in the number of private residential and nursing homes in the 1980s. Financial burden (subsidized stays in private nursing homes) could first be borne by the central government but was then shifted to local authorities. Local authorities therefore have an incentive to keep down referrals to institutions, since all costs are to be met within an overall budget covering both institutional and home care. Provider pluralism was also introduced: local authorities are not allowed to be sole providers of care but must contract out a significant proportion of both institutional and home care services to private and voluntary agencies. 'Case management' is intended to achieve needs-led provision and to overcome structural barriers between different providers.

Policy responses required: reconciling and bridging informal and formal care

Many formal home and community care systems rely on the 'backup' and 'care coordinator' services provided by informal carers. Rarely do formal home and community care services completely replace or operate in the absence of informal carers' inputs. Despite this, policies that seek to coordinate formal and family care are still extremely rare. This can be explained by the historical legacy of (in most countries) overwhelming reliance on families to deliver home care and the stark choice between family provided home care or (usually very poor quality) institutional care available to those who lacked any other alternatives.

Respite care refers to the short term placement of an older person in an institutional setting or the short term replacement of a family carer with a paid outside carer in the care recipient's home. Respite care serves the purpose of giving the informal carer a break and also possibly of providing the older person with some specialized services in the institutional setting (minor operations, nutrition advice, chiropody and so on). Community supports such as day centres, home helps, meals services, and night time and weekend caring should be more extensively available to support both older people who have informal carers and those who lack the support of family members.

Improving the quality of care is linked to improving the quality and attractiveness of care work. Somewhat surprisingly, the gender imbalance in formal care is considerably more striking than in informal care, with up to 95 percent female care workers even in supposedly 'gender equal' countries such as Sweden. The low level of financial compensation is one reason for this gender imbalance, along with the low status of care work which in turn is obviously bound up with the low pay. The 'entry level' status of much of care work is such that in many countries newly arrived migrant workers feature prominently in the sector. Rights to social protection ought to be available to all care workers, regardless of their employer or the sector they work in. It is evident that improvements in the pay of care workers would bring about positive results such as lower staff turnover which in turn would have a positive impact on the quality of care (where continuity is an important component).

Many other fundamental issues remain unresolved in debates around care locations. Which costs are taken into account when deciding whether a person should receive care at home or in an institution? What are the opportunity costs, such as, earnings and other opportunities foregone by the informal carers? What are the health costs? What are the current or future costs? How can we 'push the limits' of home care? Do new technologies have any potential to make home care easier, cheaper and more feasible even in the case of individuals with extensive care needs, or is it better to focus on the human elements of care by investing in the training and support of carers, both formal and informal? How could informal care and paid care best be combined? What level of government financial support to family carers still encourages informal care but does not demand excessive sacrifices?

The data on the coverage of services does not tell us anything about the quantity of care received by individual care recipients. Home care strategies could entail the targeting of services to those most at risk of institutionali-zation. Expanded community care might cover some people who would otherwise have ended up in nursing homes, but it might also lead to greater use of hospitals. If home and community care services become more targeted to individuals with extensive care needs, the service moves from having a 'mixed caseload' to having a 'heavy caseload' which in turn has implications for the nature and demands of care work. In short, making home care more widely available and visible may create new demands that must be met in order to ensure that the service is properly equipped.

We still know surprisingly little about what kind of care older people themselves want. It is arguable that the agenda for developing care services has been driven first and foremost by policymakers, and by financial and labour market considerations. Rarely are older people either consulted about what kind of care services they would like or, once they are in receipt of care, whether they are satisfied with it, and what kind of changes they would like to see. Such consultation and feedback are especially rare in institutional settings where it is usually taken for granted that older people are either content or incapable of expressing preferences, and that any changes requested would be excessively cumbersome and detrimental to staff working practices or even to the safety of the residents.

Conclusion

Long term care of older people is an extremely 'messy' area of research due to the large number of different services, providers and sources of funding involved. While splitting the care services into formal and informal, home/community-based and institutional does help to organize our thinking about care, these distinctions are also rather indiscriminate and increasingly blurred. For instance, an older person may be looked after in his or her own home by a relative who used to be unpaid but is now financially rewarded to some extent though a cash for care package that is also being used to hire a formal care worker in the evenings and weekends. In many countries, a shift has occurred very recently from a complete reliance on unpaid family carers to a complex mix of public, private and family care. This, in combination with the diversity of care tasks involved, ranging from personal care to housework to leisure activities and companionship results in a complex patchwork of services and benefits that has evolved gradually, and rarely as a result of any grand design.

Lack or inadequacy of home and community care, pressure on acute hospitals and the high costs and variable quality of institutional care have led policymakers in many countries to adopt a new focus on domiciliary and community care. Considerable consensus exists over the principle of enabling older persons to remain living in their own homes 'for as long as possible': however, an explanation of what exactly is meant by this is not generally provided, and the logic of the argument varies between economists, policy analysts and social workers. The thesis is often advanced that a large proportion of older persons in institutional care, provided with the right combination of services and modifications in their accommodation could in fact live in their own homes, and that the transitions from hospital or other 'medicalized' care settings into a community care setting should be accelerated, both in the interest of the care recipient and in the interest of public finances. Yet very little is known of the transitions between these care settings, of the preferences of individuals in different situations and of the kind of services and technologies that could accelerate and promote such transitions. Comprehensive financial data which would provide comparisons of the costs of institutional care vis-à-vis home care for persons at different dependency levels and with different levels of informal care support is currently lacking in most countries. Nonetheless, it is safe to say that there is a severe undersupply of domiciliary and community care services for older people in many countries, a fact that is reflected both in the heavy strain that many informal carers operate under, and by the presence in institutional care settings of many individuals whose care needs can be defined as 'low' and 'social' in nature.

While there will probably always be some older people who want and need 'medicalized' and institutional long term care, the future challenge clearly lies in developing policies that can better support older people in the location of choice of most older people, namely in their own home and community. Fortunately, there is a growing realization that home and community care are desirable from the point of view of older persons' quality of life and, where delivered in a timely manner with a focus on rehabilitation, can also serve to generate financial savings in comparison to approaches that are based on expensive and inappropriate forms of institutional care. Care preferences are powerfully shaped by the reality of the care regime: where high quality formal care is available, it becomes accepted and attractive, which in turn has the reinforcing impact of motivating people (tax payers and workers) to finance such care. In countries where such public funding mechanisms do not exist (or fund care only to the poorest), many (but by no means all) members of the future cohorts of older people will have higher incomes, more wealth and will be more consumer minded: their own choices and spending power, therefore, will become important determinants of the future of care services (Smith and Kington 1997). In the next two chapters, we will turn to discussing this and other ways in which changes in older people, younger people and policies can bring about more age friendly societies.

PART FOUR
NEW BEHAVIOURS, NEW DEMANDS, NEW CHALLENGES

9 Exercising power and challenging attitudes

Introduction

All societies have preconceptions of ageing, and a set of behavioural norms that older people are expected to adhere to, and this chapter begins with a discussion of these attitudes and expectations. In most societies, older people are expected to disengage from many mainstream adult occupations and activities. Considerable difficulties are faced by older people who wish to act outside the norms and boundaries that societies impose on them. However, these norms and behaviours are in flux: today's younger cohorts will be classified as 'older' in the future, and are likely to extend their behaviours, preferences, expectations and lifestyles into their own old age. These will in turn influence both politics and markets as older people make their choices in polling booths and supermarkets. The actual and potential influence of older people as voters, consumers and as members of interest groups is discussed. While older people are not a homogeneous group, they have nonetheless been able to form a coherent lobby group in some countries and in relation to some issues that are of central importance to them. The chapter also cautions that the differences *among* older people can be as big as the differences between older and younger people: there is therefore not a strong prospect of older people forming a 'united front' other than around areas where policies serve to generate a shared interest in preserving or strengthening them.

Perceptions of older people and attitudes towards ageing

This chapter discusses the complex issue of attitudes towards ageing. Attitudes are a very powerful determinant of older people's quality of life and also have a deep impact on policymaking. While all societies have a set of behavioural patterns and norms that older people are expected to conform to, these expectations can change over time. As circumstances, policies and individuals who occupy the 'older people' category change, attitudes can also alter.

As was pointed out in Chapter 1, there is no single 'correct' or complete definition of old age. Our sociocultural understandings of old age and ageing are the most influential interpretations of ageing, and these vary over time and across societies. Younger people's attitudes towards ageing shape the experience of ageing, but increasingly older people's changing conceptualizations of themselves and their role in society are influencing the way younger people perceive and treat them. It is important to understand how both 'younger' people and 'older' people perceive ageing and 'being old', as both sets of perceptions influence the experience of ageing.

The proliferation in the terms that refer to ageing and old age reflects the changing reality and attitudes: old age is now commonly referred to as later life, the third age, the golden years, and older people are often referred to as 'senior citizens' – all positive or neutral terms in contrast to 'elderly' or 'old people' that have come to be seen as negative and patronizing terms. In many countries older persons' organizations are campaigning for the abolition of terms such as 'elderly' and for the adoption of more neutral terms such as 'older people' or 'seniors'. Some of the relatively new terminology has a decidedly 'liberated' and 'empowered' flavour: there are references to 'grey panthers', 'super-grannies', and even members of the SKI club (which stands for 'spend-your-kids'-inheritance' – on your own leisure activities).

Ageism and other 'isms'

Various 'isms' refer to distorted representations of members of a particular group: sexism refers to treating women and men differently and racism refers to differential treatment and attitudes based on racial characteristics. Negative attitudes and discriminatory behaviours towards ageing and older people are referred to as ageism (Bytheway 1994). Ageism is systematic stereotyping and discrimination on the grounds of age. Ageism can, of course, affect young people also (for instance where an applicant is perceived to be 'too young' for a 'senior' job) but in most instances it affects older people.

Ageism is similar to sexism or racism in that it is discrimination against all members of a particular group. An ageist person or attitude views and represents older people as *different* from, and usually in some way inferior to, younger people. In the ageist worldview older people are not subject to the same wants and needs as younger people are, and can be treated differently on the grounds of their age and various negative characteristics attributed to old age. For instance, as Chapter 8 pointed out, older people are often deemed incapable of or unsuited to making decisions about their own long term care.

Ageism tends to be more covert and subtle than racism or sexism, and in many societies continues to be more accepted or tolerated than racism or sexism. Whereas the vast majority of people would now be outraged by job advertisements that stated, for instance, 'no women need apply', it is still explicitly or implicitly accepted by many that people above a certain age can be excluded from many jobs.

Stereotypes of old age and older people

Even where an attitude or a policy does not qualify as explicitly 'ageist', it can reflect stereotypical images of older people. Commonly propagated stereotypes of older people include the belief that older people are socially isolated and lonely; that they suffer from poor health; that they are a burden on younger generations; that they have no sex lives; and that they are not able to learn new skills. Unfortunately, these attitudes are sometimes held not only by younger people, but by older people themselves.

Attitudes towards ageing can be examined from three different perspectives, namely: younger people's views of old age (What 'the young' think of 'the old'); self-images of older people (how older people perceive themselves and 'being old'); and older people's views of society's attitudes towards them (how older people perceive their treatment by the rest of society).

When (predominantly young) undergraduate students taking the ageing and social policy course at my university are asked whether they can envisage the years after their sixtieth birthday as being the best years of their life, the answer is usually a bewildered 'no, of course not'. The most frequently nominated disadvantages of the later decades of life are illness, decreased mobility, poverty, loneliness, inadequate (medical) care and fear of crime. However, older people themselves consistently state that they are affected by these problems to a far lesser extent than is commonly thought. For example in the light of survey results, only a small minority of older people are deemed to be socially isolated or perceive loneliness as a problem (Chapter 3). Young students often have to reflect for a long period of time before being able to suggest any positive aspects of older age. Perhaps somewhat surprisingly (not least to the students themselves), many of the advantages that they ascribe to the later stages of the lifecycle are similar to those of youth: lack of responsibilities and a greater freedom to enjoy life (than in the overcommitted middle years of life).

How do older people perceive themselves? There is of course a wide variety of self-perceptions, some positive and others negative; however, on average they tend to be considerably more positive than perceptions by younger people of old age. For instance, according to a survey conducted by the American Association of Retired People (AARP 2002), 61 percent of men aged between 55 and 64, and 66 percent of those over the age of 65 thought that they got as much or more fun out of life as they had at a younger age. The most important aspects in the self-perception of ageing and changes in age identity are related to health, physical activity, chronological age, retirement and social roles and relationships (e.g., grandparenthood and widowhood). Self-image can remain remarkably stable over time, although (older) people also continue to construct a coherent sense of self in accordance with changed circumstances and challenges (Biggs 1999).

It is also interesting to know how older people perceive younger people's attitudes and behaviour towards themselves. An EU-wide survey undertaken in 1992 (Walker 1993) and covering the 12 countries that were members of the Union at the time involved interviews of 12,800 persons of all ages, including 5000 persons aged 60 or over. Across the EU, approximately one-third of older people felt that they had been treated with more respect as they grew older; some 60 percent agreed with the statement that younger people were helpful towards older people; over one-third reported having a lot of contact with young people; and 37 percent agreed with the statement that older people are admired and respected by younger people.

Diversity in older age

Perhaps the single most pervasive, misleading and detrimental stereotype of older people is that *they are all alike*. Researchers, too, have to bear part of the blame for this as they often treat the 65+ group as a perfectly valid group for the purposes of presenting sweeping generalizations. For instance, surveys typically base their findings on the responses from the (statistically perfectly valid and reliable) 1000 or so individuals aged 65 or over, often without highlighting the variance in the sample by gender, age, class, ethnicity or other cross-cutting cleavages. Such findings mask diversity and reinforce the popular belief that older people are a homogeneous group of people who all want the same things and think alike – often in opposition to younger people.

It cannot be denied that, considered as a group, older people often seem to share characteristics that are different from younger people. The age stratification perspective states that society makes distinctions in people's roles on the basis of age, thereby creating age strata that can be viewed much like social class in its effects. There clearly exist a large number and variety of social and legal rules and norms that enable or encourage older people to do some things, and 'disable' them in other respects. For instance, the age of 65 is a 'ticket' to retirement in many countries: people are 'free' to retire at this age. However, this could also be construed as a restriction: at the age of 65, older people must retire even if they would like to continue working. However, if we move our focus away from these socially constructed stratifications, rules and norms, what does old age in fact mean?

Age is simply an index of time, and rarely a straightforward or single *cause* of anything. First, not all older people share the same set of characteristics: there are no inevitable and inescapable characteristics that accompany old age. Second, the fact that many older people share certain characteristics does not mean that those characteristics (for instance poverty, memory loss, retirement from paid work, and so on) are *caused* by old age. Factors other than age are usually the underlying causes, and the problems associated with older age often start at a much younger age. Old age in itself does not cause either physical or social phenomena associated with ageing: for Alzheimer's disease a number of pathological processes have to take place that are more common in older age but not directly caused by older age; for poverty in old age to occur on a widespread scale society must first make decisions about allocation of resources. Third, diversity among the older population is brought about by a range of factors, many of which are attributed to the individual in childhood or even at conception or *in utero* (such as sex and aspects of personality and propensity to develop certain diseases) and continue to exert an influence throughout the individual's lifecourse.

Close readers of this book will already have identified a number of crosscutting cleavages which divide older people into diverse groups, some of which have arguably less in common with each other than 'older people' considered as a group have with 'younger people'. There are many sources of diversity among older people: some of the most important ones include gender, age ('the younger old' versus the oldest old), income and education (also referred to as socioeconomic group or social class), ethnicity, culture and health status. Location is an important differentiator too: residence in an urban or rural area, or in a deprived neighourhood, can influence the experience of old age in important ways. Chapter 4 pointed out that longevity and health status in old age vary by both gender and socioeconomic status: women live longer but experience poorer health in old age, and people from higher socioeconomic groups tend to both live longer and remain healthier than people from less economically and educationally advantaged groups. We will now briefly examine the influence of gender which has throughout the book been referred to as a central source of difference in the experience of old age.

Ageing as a gendered experience

One of the most obvious sources of difference among the older population is gender. In fact, gender is such a pervasive source of diversity in old age that the author of this book eschewed a separate chapter on 'gender and ageing' in favour of frequent references to gender throughout the book. For instance, this book has highlighted the female majorities among older cohorts, especially among the oldest old (Chapter 2), the differences in social engagement and the differential impact of marriage and divorce on older men and women (Chapter 3), and the fact that both the majority of older people and the majority of 'heavy duty' carers (in the informal *and* formal care sectors) are female (Chapters 7 and 8). Chapter 5 discussed the fact that women tend to be negatively affected by policies that are designed for the standard (male) breadwinner (such as many pension systems). This chapter also made reference to the fact that the gap between women's and men's incomes widens with age and women are more affected by old age poverty than men. Chapter 6 pointed out that many of the 'solutions' to population ageing impinge on women's lives as they tend to increasingly involve strategies to make women both have more babies *and* contribute more on the labour market.

However, it would be naive in the extreme to view all older women as having the same characteristics, experiences, needs and wishes. While gender on its own is a powerful influence on the experience of ageing, it obviously interacts with other variables such as marital status and social class (Arber et al. 2003). For instance, the old age of a widow can be very different from the later life of a married, or remarried, divorced or never married woman. Social class, which tends to translate into material well being and opportunities to make the most of the 'third age' is also a very powerful differentiator among women. Ethnicity, disability and sexual orientation also generate diversity among the older female population (Bernard et al. 2000).

It is interesting to note that until relatively recently, the attention of feminists (both inside and outside academia) focused on inequalities, discrimination and stereotyping experienced by women of working age. Older women were rarely the topic of analysis and the most prominent campaigns in the area of women's rights have been fought in areas that have not been of direct relevance for older women such as childcare, employment and reproductive rights (although it is possible that these will assume great relevance also for older women as many of them become involved in the raising of grandchildren and may also wish to work and reproduce until a much later age than has been the norm until now).

Chapter 1 discussed the difference between chronological age and social age. Social age refers to the appropriate attitudes and behaviours that society ascribes to different age groups. According to most social definitions of old age, the transition to old age happens at different stages for men and women, and the main 'rites of passage' associated with old age are quite different for women and men. Whereas retirement from paid work is a clear cut milestone and point of transition into old(er) age for many men, retirement has no real meaning for many women who, often regardless of whether they have worked outside the home or not, continue to bear the main responsibility for household management. Older women in many cases never 'retire' in any real sense of the word and tend to have less free time than men as in many cases domestic work and care (of spouse or grandchildren) continue into old age (Bernard et al. 2000). For many women, widowhood and other family events (grandparenthood or the youngest child moving away from home) are more important as markers of old age than retirement from work.

Negative attitudes towards old age tend to affect women more than men and the fact that ageism is often combined with sexism makes it particularly pernicious for women. Loss of physical attractiveness as defined by beauty ideals is often highlighted in the case of older women: women are seen to pass their 'sell by date' earlier than men. Older women are commonly depicted as worn out, unattractive, menopausal, neurotic, unproductive, 'over the hill' or even as witches. These negative perceptions may be partly rooted in the fact that, until very recently in human history, the single most valued and central 'function' of women was seen to be childbearing: once this ability is lost, woman's value is seen to diminish. In contrast, many stereotypes that are associated with older men are positive: images commonly associated with older men are being grey haired, distinguished, wise, experienced and reliable. Fortunately, the negative images of women are being eroded and counteracted by many older women who are portrayed (and choose to portray themselves) as powerful, attractive, intelligent and decisive. Of course, the situation where only good looking older women are seen as having aged successfully is a potential negative consequence of such a seemingly positive development.

Are older people powerful?

One of the great paradoxes of attitudes towards older people lies in the depiction of older people as weak and defenceless on the one hand, and as extremely powerful and influential on the other hand. For instance, Preston (1984: 445–6) has argued that

> the changing numbers of young and old have altered the environment for public policy decisions. In a modern democracy, public decisions are obviously influenced by the power of special interest groups, and that power is in turn a function of the size of the groups, the wealth of the groups, and the degree to which that size and wealth can be mobilized for concerted action. In all of these areas, interests of the elderly have gained relative to those of children.

Contrast this with the frequent alerts in the media to poverty, appalling housing conditions, abuse, fear of crime and even malnutrition among older people, and the paradox is ready. We appear to have a rather 'schizophrenic' view of older people as influential and dominant (to the detriment of other population groups) on the one hand and as victims on the other hand.

Does the increase in the number of older voters and in interest representation on behalf of older people mean that they are able to wield more political power? We now turn to discussing the factors that seem to increase the political influence of older people, and those that counteract such a development.

There are two main ways in which older people (or indeed anyone) can seek to influence public policies: as voters or as members of interest groups. A number of factors appear to strengthen the potential of older people to influence policy. In a democracy, everyone has one vote: the more people in a given group with common interests and shared preferences for how and by whom those interests should be served, the greater their power to influence the outcome of elections (electoral systems obviously play a powerful role in translating votes into seats in the representative bodies, but for now we are working on the assumption of straightforward proportional representation). A very large and growing number of older voters now exists in many developed countries, and assuming that they all, or a majority of them, vote for the same party or parties that effectively represent their interests, they will become a political force to be reckoned with. As the proportion of older people in the population increases, the 'grey vote' becomes more desirable for politicians, especially as in many countries a large proportion of older people vote (in contrast to widespread voter apathy among young adults in particular). Interest groups for older people have also proliferated in many countries, and there are even international organizations (for example at the European Union level) that seek to improve older people's position across a large number of countries (Walker and Naegele 1999).

However, there are a number of obstacles to what is sometimes portrayed as an inexorable rise in the political power of older people. The most obvious obstacle is the fact that not all older people vote for the same party or group of parties that specialize(s) or would be forced to specialize in promoting older people's interests. Cohesiveness of attitudes and voting among older people is relatively weak compared to cohesiveness among classes, races or religions (Manza and Brooks 1999). It has also been shown that wealthy voters, including wealthy older voters, tend to vote against social protection policies as a whole, rather than for policies for older people and against policies for children (Brooks and Brady 1999). Most people develop party loyalty at a relatively young age and do not shift their allegiance easily. Therefore, the fact that older people vote for a certain party may be a cohort effect (people who have always voted for that party entering old age) rather than a shift by older voters to favour that party.

Despite these caveats, it is demonstrably the case that politicians sometimes do pursue the 'grey vote', particularly where older people are seen as having the potential to act as swing voters in tightly contested elections or electoral districts. For example, as part of the 2007 Australian election campaign, the incumbent government in its last pre-election budget allocated a US$500 one off payment to all older people. This was widely seen as an attempt to demonstrate older-people-friendly credentials and also to swing the older vote in favour of the government in some marginal seats (the incumbents lost).

In many countries older people's interest groups are rather small and fragmented and have no demonstrable impact on public policy. A notable exception is the American Association of Retired People (AARP 2007) that has some 38 million members. A number of international organizations for older people have also come into existence, for instance at the European level, but these tend to be more focused on general issues campaigns than targeted policy campaigns. The structure of entitlements is a very powerful influence on the success of attempts to rally older voters around a cause: where all or most older people are entitled to the same pensions and healthcare, they are more likely to defend their benefits and services successfully. Conversely, where the structure of policies and entitlements divides older people into constituencies that have different interests, cutback attempts are more likely to succeed: a good example are the pension reforms in the UK in the 1980s (see Chapter 5).

In conclusion, it would certainly be naive to portray older people as a cohesive political force: older people, by and large, divide their political allegiances between parties, as does the rest of the population. It is also erroneous to portray older people as exclusively focused on their own issues. Most people are long termist, consistent and broad in their affective and practical support for different generations as they usually have close relatives who belong to these different age groups. People rarely vote for 'the young people's party' or 'the old people's party' but rather for parties that they have come to favour through the overall attractiveness of their agendas and approaches. In fact, it is difficult to think of parties that would have chosen to style themselves as older people's parties (and the ones that have, have tended to remain very marginal or disappear completely). Often, the parties that are 'generous' to older people are also generous to younger people, in other words, they have general redistributive agendas. It has to be acknowledged, however, that their growing number and tendency to use their vote and ability to sometimes swing the vote in marginal constituencies can 'play into the hands' of older voters. Political parties may also seek to entice older voters especially in elections where they are perceived to be the critical constituency; however, it is not older persons' 'fault' if parties seek to garner favour in this way. Indeed, it should be seen as democracy in action.

Influence through non-political channels

Politics is not the only way, and arguably not even the most powerful way, of influencing perceptions and experience of old age. New cohorts of older people are constantly bringing new behaviours and expectations into their old age. Many of the so-called 'baby-boomers' in particular are determined to change the face of ageing. It is reasonable to surmise, for instance, that many of these 'new older people' will (where sufficient pension or other wealth is available to them) maintain 'consumerist' lifestyles (Pebley 1998). This, in turn, would serve to counteract the belief that consumer spending is inevitably suppressed as a result of population ageing. On the negative side, such behaviours could add to environmental problems. However, it is also possible that older people's extended co-existence with grandchildren will make them more conscious of the long term impact of their purchasing decisions and therefore more ecologically aware as consumers. Older people's consumer behaviours are as unpredictable and as much subject to future change as any other group's behaviour (Harper 2006).

Outside their role as voters or consumers, too, older adults may choose to engage, in increasing numbers, in behaviours that are today seen as outrageous. For instance, recent years have seen several high profile cases of women in their sixties giving birth to babies following in vitro fertilizations and closely monitored pregnancies. One such mother (with four other children from an earlier phase of life) challenged her critics: 'I don't feel like 60. I don't know what 60 is supposed to be'. To counter the horror of some people at such behaviour, it bears pointing out that an educated, healthy, well to do woman in her early sixties has a lengthy (healthy) remaining life expectancy, the economic resources and, clearly, the determination and probably the emotional reserves to see the child reach adulthood. Why do we consider her less acceptable as a parent than a younger person (male or female) who may lack all or most of these characteristics? The tastes, preferences and lifestyles of older people are diverse and continually evolving, and will require changes in attitudes on the part of younger people.

Conclusion

While older people are not a very homogeneous group, they have nonetheless been able to form a fairly coherent lobby group in a number of countries and in relation to a number of issues that are of central importance to them. It is increasingly evident that politicians are mindful of the increasing numbers of older voters and their propensity to vote (although not necessarily for any party that makes promises to them, party preferences in many cases having been formed at younger ages and being unlikely to change quickly). The most attitude transforming influence of older people, however, is likely to take place by virtue of their private choices as individuals regarding their lifestyles and consumption patterns. These are continually changing as new cohorts enter old age and bring with them new behaviours and expectations.

10 Conclusion: what will the 'silver century' look like?

Introduction

This chapter concludes the book with a discussion of the ways in which societies are striving to strike a balance between cost and fairness considerations in their attempts to adapt to population ageing. While much remains to be done, particularly in the area of transforming attitudes towards ageing, considerable reform activity in the area of old age policies is already evident in many countries. While some of these policies have the character of retrenchment (e.g., some aspects of pensions reforms), others are genuinely new and represent social policy expansion, recalibration and improvement. Ageing and old age policies are in a state of constant flux, are connected to a wide range of social and political developments and phenomena, and as such constitute a rich field for future work and analysis. It is increasingly imperative that this analysis adopts a genuinely inter-disciplinary approach as it is only through understanding the relationships between health, socio-economic status and social engagement of older individuals that effective policies can be designed.

Ageing – a great human achievement

Ageing is a success, a great achievement, and should be treated first and foremost as a positive phenomenon. People live longer, and in large parts of the world old age is healthier, wealthier and arguably even happier than in the past. Previously most lives consisted of childhood and (for those who survived the perilous early stages of life) a long period spent in (re)productive work, followed immediately or fairly closely by death. Now a new stage has been added to people's lives and, in developed countries (and increasingly also in developing countries), we are likely to reach that stage. In addition to childhood, youth and work, an extended period of leisure precedes death for most people in the developed world. It cannot be denied that this combination of longer, healthier and financially more secure old age is one of the great, and possibly the greatest, achievements of humankind (while acknowledging, of course, that a healthy and secure old age is still far from a universal phenomenon).

Population ageing is a complex phenomenon that cannot and should not be stopped or reversed. The earlier chapters in this book were devoted to examining both the prerequisites for and implications of population ageing, that is to say the changes in society, economy, gender roles and personal behaviours that contributed towards bringing about the phenomenon of ageing, and that are needed to adapt to ageing. Obviously, in the face of such extensive and powerful socioeconomic developments, governments can do little to stop population ageing. A number of countries have attempted to slow down the rate of population ageing by offering incentives to child-bearing, but these have had no or only rather marginal impact. On the balance of the results of such attempts to date, we cannot, and probably should not, combat ageing, but we can and should try to ensure that the experience of ageing becomes more positive both for older people and for societies as a whole. To this end, a large number of inter-linked changes in policy, practices and attitudes are needed.

Despite the obvious significance of population ageing, most societies today are preoccupied with youth, or with youthfulness. Investment in children and young people is frequently stressed, and numerous government reports and scholarly projects have been devoted to examining the improvements in children's rights and policies targeted to children. These are naturally welcome and desirable developments, but they do sometimes contrast starkly with lesser concern with older people. There are many reasons why a similar development is yet to take place in older people's rights and services in many countries, but it is safe to say that we are witnessing an increasing interest in older people, across the globe, on the part of both politicians and policymakers and the scholarly community. The adaptations required at the level of policies and practices towards older people are even more extensive, and daunting for many.

A difficult question: how should societies change as a result of ageing?

It is clear that both individuals and societies are yet to fully adapt to ageing. Despite the solid fact of extended lives, we still tend to have a 'compressed' view of our lifetime where key achievements must be reached by the age of 30 or 40, instead of 50 or 60. For instance, despite the fact that a young (in particular an educated and wealthy) woman can now reasonably expect to live to 85 or 90 in many countries, and to work until her late sixties or even seventies, many women delay or forego motherhood because of the perceived necessity to devote their reproductive age to building their career. If there existed both the realization at the individual level that a woman in her early thirties will have several decades left to further her career and the facilitation at the societal and policy level of breaks from work and (working) mother-hood in general, fewer women might decide to forego motherhood (it is possible, of course, that even such 'calculations' and policy measures would not trump over the preference for other 'goods' in life such as time and ability to develop as an individual in other arenas of life).

This book concludes with a discussion of the ways in which societies are striving to strike a balance between cost and fairness considerations in their attempts to improve the quality of life of older people while bearing in mind resource constraints. This chapter flags and briefly discusses some of the highly important policy and practical questions that are growing in salience as populations age: should older people work longer? Should they be given access to more and better medical treatment and greater choice in their own care, including possibly the right to terminate their lives in case of terminal illnesses? Why should we invest more in older people and their quality of life? All these questions have in common the fact that, to a very great extent, our answers to them are bound up with our attitudes to ageing and older people.

Ageist policies and practices

Many policies and practices are infused with ageism. The following are some examples of ageist policies and practices.

In the area of *heathcare and medical treatments*, older people are frequently assumed to be less deserving of medical treatment than younger patients (see Chapter 4). Many healthcare professionals tend to dismiss health complaints in older people as being a natural and unavoidable part of old age. A frequent response to health complaints by older people is: 'there is nothing that can be done about it, it is just due to old age'. Older patients can be refused treatment or made to wait longer because of their age. Prescribing practices among doctors may also discriminate against older patients: whereas more advanced or more expensive treatments and medications are given to younger patients, older people are more likely to be offered inferior drugs (Huebschmann et al. 2006). Even pain relief is sometimes not prescribed for older adults due to the ingrained belief that old age simply is miserable. In reality, there are many different ways of curing or at least significantly alleviating conditions that are common in older people.

Ageism in service delivery is illustrated by the fact that older persons' services are rarely rehabilitative in nature: instead of seeking to restore abil-ities, they are normally designed to enable the older person to 'get by'. For instance, whereas a younger person may be provided with intensive rehabi-litation to restore the ability to walk and thereby manage their own shopping and other chores, an older person would more commonly be provided with a home help or similar service that does the shopping on her behalf. The rehabilitative and activating approach may sometimes be more expensive in the short term, but results in savings in the longer term: it is frequently assumed that the remaining lifespan in older people is not sufficient to garner back the costs of such investment. Healthcare for older people is often overmedicalized as it is assumed that medicines, and not rehabilitation or social supports, are the best method of taking care of (suppressing) health needs in older people. This is also reflected in the lack or poor availability of services that address the social and psychological needs of older people.

Another example of ageism is the compulsory screening of people because they have reached a certain age or failing to screen them because they are over a certain age limit. For instance, in many countries free breast cancer screening is limited to 50–65-year-olds, although over sixty-fives can also develop breast cancer. Older drivers over a specific age limit are in some countries required to take a new driving test before their licence is renewed or to undergo compulsory medical tests despite the lack of any conclusive evidence that such compulsory testing reduces accidents or that older people are dangerous drivers. The fact that older drivers are involved in more fatal accidents than middle aged drivers is largely attributable to the fact that older drivers are frailer and hence more likely to be killed in a crash (Loughran and Seabury 2007). Older drivers tend to drive shorter distances, stay off motorways, avoid driving at night and are on the whole more cautious than younger drivers.

The lack or inadequacy of quality controls in *long term* care services for older people reflects the attitude that different, less exacting standards apply to older people than to children for example (see Chapter 8). Lack of consultation of patients regarding their daily routines is generally accepted practice in institutional care and many other areas of service provision. Older people are viewed as being passive recipients of services, who are incapable of exercising informed choice over their own lives. There is a tendency to equate older people with children ('infantalization' of older people).

Examples of deep rooted and widely accepted ageism are also rife in the areas of *employment* and *education*. While overt discrimination on the grounds of age in the recruitment of workers may be prohibited, in practice many employers are not prepared to consider employees above a certain age. Imposing a compulsory retirement age on older workers can be seen as a form of discrimination, on rather absurd grounds: how does one suddenly become unfit to work or undesirable as an employee after one's sixty-fifth birthday? Education and retraining opportunities often exclude older people because it is assumed that they cannot absorb new information or acquire new skills, or will not be working sufficiently long or productively for society and/or employers to benefit from these skills. The issue of compulsory retirement ages is a complex one that will be discussed in detail below. Current retirement ages are universally acknowledged to be rather arbitrary, yet their usage is persistent. In many countries older workers are not covered by employment rights legislation to the same extent as employees under the age of 65. If we are to take the ambition of extending working lives seriously, new policies have to be developed that give greater individual choice in when to retire, and more incentives for employers to hire and retain older workers.

Even many commonly held beliefs about incomes in older age can be profoundly ageist. It is often implicitly or explicitly argued that studying older people's living standards in the light of their incomes alone is inappropriate. After all, in many countries older people have access to resources that are unavailable to working age population, or at least cost more for younger people than for older people. First and foremost, home ownership rates are very high among older people in many countries: whereas younger people are still paying their mortgages, older people are free from this often significant financial burden. Healthcare is in many countries free or cheaper for older people than for people of working age. Free or subsidized transport services may be made available to older citizens. Older people also tend to have fewer work related expenses, as they do not need to travel to work every day, purchase 'work clothes' and so on.

It is therefore often argued that, taking into account the broader picture (assets, services, lifestyle), older people are in fact rather well off and not in need of any improvements in their incomes. There are a number of reasons for rejecting this argument. First, while older people are in some countries 'asset rich', they can also be very 'cash poor' due to low pension incomes. This frequently leads to a situation where they are unable to afford the modifications or renovation work that are necessary in order to make their homes more suitable or comfortable. In other words, many older people are forced to 'run down' the main asset that they own, and may find themselves in cold or damp accommodation, or even unable to use parts of the house (e.g., rooms upstairs) due to mobility problems. Second, while older people often pay less than people in younger age groups towards their housing and healthcare, and are not affected by work related expenses or childcare expenses, their needs in other areas may increase. Poor health or mobility problems can necessitate the purchase of medicines, devices and services (including care) that are not always covered by the welfare state. Third, it is unfair to assume that older people do not 'need' as much money as younger people 'because they are happy sitting at home watching TV and eating biscuits' in contrast to following the more exciting and expensive leisure pursuits of younger people. It is frequently assumed that all older people have similar preference for inexpensive, sedate lifestyles – whereas in reality their aspirations in this area vary and have increased considerably in recent decades.

In addition to income poverty, social exclusion also affects many older people. Social exclusion arises where individuals are prevented from taking part in activities that are seen as the norm, or as 'rights' for the rest of the population. Social exclusion differs from poverty in that it is not always the result of low income alone. For instance, older people can be socially excluded because they lack opportunities to participate in mainstream activities such as employment and education; because they are made to feel unwelcome in pubs or clubs; or because they lack suitable transport and other services. A national British study (Patsios 2000) found pensioners at risk of being excluded from social relations, which were operationalized in terms of non-participation in common social activities, as a result of unaffordability or unavailability, social isolation, lack of social support, civic disengagement and confinement due to physical ill health. In order to address social exclusion, a combination of improved incomes (particularly for disadvantaged older people such as some groups of older women) and changed attitudes and opportunity structures is required.

Why does ageism persist? What can be done to eliminate it?

Stereotypes about older people, women, ethnic minorities, etc. are a shorthand method of communicating the social value of specific social groups and influence our social interaction with them by suggesting appropriate forms of behaviour. There are many causes of ageism, including a deep rooted fear of growing old – a stage of life that people commonly associate with the loss of independence, loss of mobility, loss of income and loss of many loved ones – in other words, multiple losses of the things that many people value most highly in life. In contrast, many cultures have come to put increasing value on youth which is associated with independence, fulfilling work, beauty, strength and exciting life experiences.

We will now turn to a discussion of one of the most controversial, yet crucial debates that have arisen as a result of population ageing: should older people be made to retire later, in other words, should working lives be extended in the light of the mounting costs of pensions and improved health status of older people? Somewhat paradoxically (and certainly controversially), answering, 'yes', to this question may prove to be one of the most significant steps towards a less ageist society, if planned and implemented properly.

Should working lives be extended?

Changing entrenched practices and expectations around retirement is a controversial and complex issue. The opportunity to retire at 65 is seen by many as an important right that has been achieved after a long struggle, and that should not be easily surrendered. It is also evident that the will to retire does not always co-exist with the ability to retire. However, this is further complicated, especially in the case of manual workers, by the problem that the capacity to undertake some tasks can decline over time, necessitating retraining. This group of workers, in particular, is then affected by the assumption that older people cannot acquire new skills and so should be removed from the workplace. It also has to be acknowledged that socio-economic and occupational differences serve to bring about differences in the ability (and willingness) to work until an older age: a compulsory increase in retirement ages across the board could have the adverse effect of enabling those who are in good health and in interesting and well paid jobs having the opportunity to further improve their financial situation, while those most in need of pensions and least capable of carrying on working without assistance being forced to continue to work, even when their capacity has declined and expected period of benefiting from pensions is shorter than those of the healthier and better off workers. It is clearly not easy to balance the right to retire at 65 and the right to continue working after 65. The main 'pros', 'cons' and challenges of the drive to extend working lives are summarized in Box 10.1 below.

Box 10.1   Extending working lives

1   *Pros*:

- involvement in central sphere of valued social and economic activity;
- transforming one major method of excluding older adults from mainstream activity;
- addressing fears of those concerned with costs of pensions;
- tapping into the reservoir of talent and ability in the older population.

2   *Cons*:

- equity considerations: socioeconomic differences in life expectancy, health and occupational profiles;
- possible reduction in older persons' involvement in other valuable spheres, e.g., voluntary sector.

3   *Challenges*:

- developing retraining and rehabilitation services, and life-long learning;
- transforming employer attitudes;
- convincing those who have a strong preference for leisure over income;
- enabling work where possible and desirable, allowing retirement (including early retirement) where necessary.

An additional year of employment represents a proportionately greater loss of time spent in retirement for those with shorter life expectancies. Socioeconomic inequalities tend to be exacerbated in old age, and the class divide matters in old age even more than it does at younger age. The experience, and even the duration of 'old age' varies by socioeconomic class. The results of the English Longitudinal Study of Ageing (ELSA) indicate that on average, people in the highest socioeconomic class live around five years longer than people in the lowest socioeconomic class and that the richest and highest educated sections of society begin to experience mental and physical disabilities on average 15 years later than people in the lowest social group (Banks et al. 2006). Even in the world of increasing longevity, this is a very long period in favour of the better off. In the US, the Health and Retirement Study (HRS) showed that the mortality rates of white males with the highest levels of education were 10 percent lower than the mortality rates of white males with the lowest education level in 1960; by 1990–97 this difference had increased to 70 percent.

People who are working in pleasant surroundings, in high status, highly remunerated jobs that are often very interesting and challenging, are understandably more inclined to continue working than those in boring, exhausting and badly paid jobs with no challenges and little social interaction. According to a US study, 57 percent of chief executives retained an office in their company for at least two years after retirement in contrast to 23 percent of senior managers (Sonnenfeld). Among the early retirees, there are currently many 'fortunate' ones who have been able to retire due to sufficient material security and interest in avenues other than their work, and the 'unfortunate' ones who have to leave work due to ill health or occupational hazards or want to leave work because it is highly unpalatable (Quinn et al. 1998).

While very few studies have been carried out to explore the complex area of retirement preferences, many older people approach the idea of working longer rather unenthusiastically, except where the possibility to combine work and leisure exists. There are major challenges in persuading *employers* to change their attitudes towards older workers. Many employers remain to be convinced to hire and retain older workers. Governments, it appears, are the only ones that are genuinely enthusiastic about the prospect of delaying retirement. Despite this, they often continue to create incentives for shedding older workers, and can be very slow to offer incentives for retaining, recruiting and retraining them. For instance, offering older workers early retirement can be the only or main channel of unloading surplus staff created by labour laws (this has been a common practice in Japan and Germany). Policies that are designed to protect employees can also have the unintended consequence of fostering employer reticence in employing older workers: for instance, if health insurance costs and pension contributions are considerably higher for an older than for a younger worker, employers will be drawn to employing younger people. Mechanisms for equalizing such costs should be developed so that employers are not penalized for hiring or retaining older workers.

Quite apart from the use of older people opportunistically as a reserve labour force, many employers have come to appreciate their reliability, loyalty, punctuality, customer-friendliness and other positive characteristics. The productivity of older workers (aged 55 and over) has been shown to be equal to, and in some cases even higher, than younger workers' productivity, even in the manufacturing sector that is often thought to require the characteristics that are usually associated with youth (strength and stamina) (Hellerstein et al. 1999). Older age is an advantage in many jobs requiring brainpower and experience. Older workers also tend to have lower rates of absenteeism than younger ones. Despite these positive attributes, employers tend to be reluctant to invest in older workers as they assume that they will be able to derive a return for their investment for a shorter time than in the case of younger workers. However, this is often an erroneous assumption as older workers tend to be more loyal and less likely to switch jobs than younger workers. The convention of seniority pay makes older workers more expensive than younger ones, but their experience may compensate for their higher cost.

As Chapter 5 pointed out, older people's attitudes towards working in later life vary considerably in line with the generosity of pensions. In countries with low pensions and incomplete pension coverage, at least some sections of the older population will have to work simply in order to earn an adequate income, as their pensions are too low to protect them against poverty or to enable them to purchase necessary and desirable goods and services. Such a situation is undesirable for a number of reasons, including the fact that those least able to work on health grounds are under the greatest pressure to do so on economic grounds (Chapter 4). The gap between rich and poor pensioners has already widened in some countries as a result of pension reforms, for instance where privatization of pension systems has been substantial (such as in the UK). In devising the future strategies for extending working lives, it is of utmost importance to bear in mind that cuts in pensions and increased reliance on private pensions and work income can lead to greater inequality in access to retirement and retirement incomes. Future reforms must be designed to enable retirement where necessary, retraining where possible and continuation of employment where possible and desirable.

Although at present we have only limited evidence of whether strategies for delaying retirement work, it is likely that the recent pension reforms and incentives to work longer will bring about a gradual and probably rather modest increase in the average age of retirement in the developed contries.

The Nordic countries have gone furthest in developing policies to allow gradual retirement and while it is as yet too early to conclusively establish their effectiveness, the early indications are promising. Demographic and economic developments may also bring about a renewed interest in older workers. As the workforce shrinks in many countries, employers and governments may become more focused on developing strategies for attracting older people back to work. This will involve offering more flexible contracts, for instance the opportunity to work part time. Where retirees have to work in order to secure a decent income and where the labour market is tighter, older workers often have to accept lower pay if they wish to remain employed or to be hired. In Japan, companies typically retire workers at 55 or 60 and then re-hire some of them at 50–70 percent of their previous pay.

These policies and developments have to be placed in the context of acknowledging that many people have a strong preference for free time over higher pensions and incomes. The range of entertainment that is available to people in old age is wider, and the cost of this entertainment is relatively lower than before. Foreign travel and home entertainment are within the financial means of most retired people in the developed countries. Many (older) people have a strong preference for a unit of free time over a unit of income: for instance, survey evidence indicates that in France people prefer early retirement to a higher pension. However, preferences stated in surveys are not always borne out by actual behaviour. Most older people would prefer a combination of work *and* leisure, rather than one or the other (McGivern 2001), and it is reasonable to expect that both employers and pension systems will increasingly facilitate such a combination of work (pay) and retirement (pension). In addition to income, employment offers other, non-material rewards. Employment can provide companionship and social engagement, and foster the sense of belonging that are important for health and well being (Chapter 3). Stimulus and companionship are welcome for many older people, and especially men who are more used to making social contacts at work and whose self-esteem is built on the basis of their work roles.

The importance of opportunities for retraining and moving to a different set of tasks within or outside an organization cannot be overemphasized. For obvious reasons, older workers tend to be in 'older' occupations that are also more strenuous and stressful than 'newer' jobs that are predominantly held by younger people. If extending working lives is taken seriously, older workers must be given the time and financial security to retrain in order to acquire tasks that are more feasible and more attractive for them. Table 10.1 summarizes these and other policy tools and challenges that are involved in the process of extending working lives.

The emphatic but heavily qualified answer to the question posed at the start of this section is therefore, 'yes, working lives should be extended'. In many countries, early exit from work, enforced retirement ages, low pensions

Table 10.1 Summary of policy tools and challenges involved in extending working lives

Current status	Aim of active ageing policies	Policy tools	Challenges
Retired	Return to work.	Creating financial incentives; offering retraining and rehabilitation where necessary.	Modest financial incentives not sufficient to entice (better off) pensioners back to work; initial cost of retraining or rehabilitation.
Working	Stay in work.	Create financial incentives to work longer, e.g., higher pension accrual rates; re-training necessary for some groups.	Those with interesting jobs and those with poor pension prospects may stay on regardless; attraction of leisure may be greater than attraction of extra pension income.
Home duties	Take up work.	Offering pensions even to late and short term entrants to paid employment; offering the possibility of combining pensions and income from work.	If no recent work history and qualification, likely to be offered only unskilled jobs; pension accrual may be modest; may not have time to work outside home!

and prejudice against hiring older workers conspire to bring about a fall in incomes in later life (Townsend 1981). Even in countries with better pensions provision, older workers are frequently squeezed out of the workplace as a result of various push and pull factors. This situation could be changed with the help of legislation to outlaw age discrimination, better work opportunities for older people including flexible working patterns, incentives for employers to hire and retain older workers, and better pensions for those who have to retire. Fulfilling the aim of active ageing may not require investing more (in fact the ultimate aim seems to be to spend less), but it does call for investing differently: in retraining, life-long learning, occupational mobility (making sure people don't get stuck in unrewarding and exhausting jobs) and enabling the combination of work and retirement.

This chapter argues that increasing the average age of retirement is not an inherently negative or undesirable development. As life expectancies are increasing almost everywhere, it is not unreasonable to strive to increase the average age of exit from employment as the number of years in retirement has increased significantly and workers can still look forward to several years of retirement even if they retire later than the previous generation. However, the significant intra-generational inequalities in health status, income, quality of work and life expectancy pose a major challenge for policymakers. While the average life expectancy has increased significantly almost everywhere, these gains in the length of life are rather unevenly distributed so that the lower socioeconomic groups have made considerably more modest gains than the better off.

Retirement from paid work is an unambiguous change of role which indicates a shift from economic independence to financial dependence. This is a crucial transition in societies which are strongly influenced by notions of economic independence and productivity. It is arguable that withdrawal (compulsory or voluntary) from paid work contributes indirectly, but nonetheless strongly, to negative attitudes towards older people in societies where productivity and being economically active have come to be seen as major indicators of social value. While the drive to extend working lives is not an unqualifiedly positive enterprise (see Chapter 5 for a discussion of the potential impact of extending working lives), it is possible to interpret it as anti-ageist. As older workers are stripped of the right to retire early, their dependence on income sources other than paid work is delayed, and thereby the perception of older people as dependent is lessened. Somewhat paradoxically, lengthening working lives (if done correctly, i.e., by taking the policy steps outlined above) may turn out to be a highly positive development from the point of view of improving attitudes towards older people and their overall status and well being in society. There is a danger, of course, that such a development may contribute to even deeper discrimination of older people who are outside the labour force for a variety of reasons (Bytheway et al. 2007). However, if extensions in working life are carried out with the above cautions in mind, and in parallel with improvements in supports for those who need them, such a danger can be minimized.

Acknowledging diversity and accepting new behaviours

Chapter 1 highlighted the fact that in addition to the quantitative aspects of ageing that are so often highlighted, ageing has very important qualitative aspects: there are more older people, but they are also doing different things and thinking differently than older people did in the past. Many older people choose to live very differently from the previous generations of older people. They have an interest in travelling or returning to education, they are working longer than expected and they may even choose to lead lives that are not very different from those led by much younger individuals. Most older people today are fitter, healthier, richer and arguably happier than older people were in the past.

Older people's status and lifestyles are constantly changing, and language plays a very important role in this process of change: terms such as 'old people', 'elderly people', 'older people' and 'senior citizens' have different connotations and therefore they influence the way we approach ageing and older people. Current stereotypes about ageing teach us to ignore, fear and detest the old, as they are portrayed as a non-productive and dependent group within societies, which (for the most part) place most value on economic productivity and independence. As well as influencing our behaviour towards the target group, stereotypes communicate appropriate forms of behaviour to the groups themselves. Modern stereotypes of ageing inform older persons that successful ageing is best achieved either by invisibility, and gratitude for the benefits which are given to them by the rest of society, or by the extension of 'youthful' behaviours and characteristics into old age.

Admittedly, even many of the analytical tools, concepts, research questions and statistical terms that are commonly employed to measure and understand ageing have in-built ageist assumptions: for instance, the term 'dependency ratios' implies that older people are dependent on the rest of society and that they therefore create a burden that has to be managed at a great cost to younger generations (Chapter 6).

We are constantly bombarded by conflicting images of older people. The images of frail, poor, sickly and powerless older people exist side by side with images of happy and healthy 'seniors' making the most of their 'third age'. Campaigns tend to focus on 'successful' older people who have managed to stay in employment, achieving very senior positions and remaining youthful. These images and expectations might contribute to policies shifting in the direction of 'active ageing', in other words, the promotion of strategies that aim to keep older people in the workforce for as long as possible. It is, of course, important to offer older people choices in all areas of life, including employment, but it is equally important to acknowledge that not all older people have similar capacities, and that certain sections of the older population need extensive care services. It is rather absurd to advocate 'positive ageing' to an older population that contains many people living in poor health, poverty and without access to the health and social care services that they need. Indeed, excessive highlighting of 'positive' or 'active' ageing in such contexts can have the (unintended) consequence of turning attention away from the very serious policy issues that should be tackled in order to ensure that more older people have a chance of having a positive ageing experience. Instead of completely rejecting or overly enthusiastically embracing either the 'negative' or 'positive' images, it makes sense to accept that they reflect different sides of the multifarious experience of old age in modern societies.

Creating an age friendly society

As various chapters in this book have highlighted, older people in many countries continue to experience both systematic discrimination in many areas of life, such as employment and healthcare, and are disadvantaged by negative attitudes towards older people. Ageism is so ingrained and embedded in social norms and practices that it is evident not only in the wider society and many professionals working with older people, but among large sections of the older population too.

The actual impact of physiological and other changes associated with ageing is highly dependent on the environment in which individuals age which includes not only the climate of attitudes that surrounds them but also the availability and quality of supports and services. In a striking example of supporting an older person, the late Pope John Paul II was able to remain in his role until death despite severe disabilities. It is obvious that similar efforts are not made in the case of the vast majority of older people. In most countries, services and supports need to be considerably expanded and improved before older people can reach their fullest potential and have the best possible quality of life.

It is sometimes said that the twentieth century was a period of rapid improvement in the lives and rights of children, and that a similar enhancement will take place in older people's position in society in the twenty-first century. The exact policy challenges differ between countries: some have made considerable progress towards ensuring income security, good service provision and equal rights in employment and other areas of life for older people, whereas in others policy is non-existent or relies on services that are not specifically designed for an ageing population.

That societies should invest in children is perceived as a foregone conclusion. The idea of 'investing in older people' appears absurd to many who assume that such investment could never 'pay off'. However, there are many reasons why societies should 'invest' in older people, too. Indeed, the creation of an age friendly society yields many benefits for all age groups and should appear attractive to younger persons in light of the fact that they are highly likely to reach old age themselves.

For instance, pensions are usually seen as transfer payments that are a burden on the rest of the population and are given primarily for reasons of inter-generational solidarity, poverty reduction or income maintenance. This portrayal of pensions as being a mechanism primarily for maintaining older persons' incomes at an acceptable level and honouring pre-existing commitments disguises the more dynamic functions that pensions can serve. As has been pointed out in Chapter 5, pensions are increasingly designed to act as work incentives: the longer you work, the more pension you earn. The guarantee of what is perceived as a good pension can therefore provide incentives for people to work longer and to be more productive. In this sense, workers 'investing' in a pension can bring about extensive benefits for economies and populations as a whole. Chapters 6 and 7 have pointed out that most services for older people continue to operate on the principle of meeting older people's needs rather than enabling them to regain their abilities. Investment in rehabilitation has the potential to yield major gains in life quality for older people, as well as long term cost savings. Investing in older people can also help families, especially women. If older people have adequate independent incomes and access to supports they are in a better position to lead independent lives, opting for services that *they* deem desirable and suitable. Adequate pensions and care are not only an insurance for older people against the risk of not being able to work or look after themselves, but also for working age people whose parents are old and frail.

It is also important to acknowledge that there are hidden, unacknowledged forms of 'active ageing'. Older people's contributions to society are numerous, but often 'invisible'. Chapters 3 and 8 have highlighted the fact that a significant proportion of informal carers are older, yet their important contributions are usually ignored. In countries that have weak social services provision, older carers of both children and older people enable labour market participation of others (e.g., the parents of the grandchildren they look after) and also enable the government to forego significant amounts of expenditure (although the opportunity costs for the carers themselves are obviously high). In the voluntary sector, too, older people are often underpinning the operation of valuable services targeted at younger and older population groups.

Inter-disciplinary approach to ageing

Well being and quality of life in old age are complex notions and their meaning varies greatly between individuals and societies. However, it stands to reason (and research has shown) that life quality and well being are dependent on a number of health related, social and economic factors (Rowe and Kahn 1999; Bond and Corner 2004; Walker and Hagan Hennessy 2004; Bowling 2005; Walker 2005). The fact that well being is dependent on many different facets of life should be reflected in the approach taken to ageing research. Greater cooperation between ageing specialists from different academic disciplines and professions is necessary if the experience of ageing is to be understood and if successful interventions are to be designed. For instance, while there is plentiful evidence that social engagement has a beneficial impact on longevity and health, there is insufficient evidence on the extent to which this applies to older populations across the world, and on whether the direction of the 'causal arrow' (from health to social engagement, or from social engagement to health) changes over the lifecourse (for instance it is possible that social engagement influences health up to a certain age, after which health begins to exert a stronger influence on social engagement). If we had a better understanding of the exact mechanisms involved and the direction of causation between health and social aspects of people's lives, more effective interventions could be designed (if health determines levels of social engagement, it clearly makes sense to invest in healthcare but if social engagement drives health, investment in social interventions makes more sense). To express the same point in broader terms, once a more profound understanding of what constitutes and contributes to 'good old age' has been achieved, policy stands a better chance of modifying the central factors. While it stands to reason that ill health, poverty and isolation are not conducive to happy old age, research can play a central role in establishing the magnitude (and cost) of such adverse effects, and also in highlighting the inter-connectedness of such negative aspects of some older people's lives. For instance, it is easier to argue for services that are currently seen by many policymakers as luxuries if it can be shown that they have measurable positive impacts on, say, the mental health of older persons, which in turn can lead to reduced institutional care costs and increased labour market participation and community engagement.

Conclusion

This book has addressed the demographics of population ageing, the family and social contexts of growing older, the health status of older populations, work and pensions as sources of income in old age, community and institutional long term care, attitudes towards older people, and the policy and practical changes that are needed at individual and societal levels in order to adapt to ageing. The book has sought to highlight the fact that almost everything that we study in the area of ageing is both a *de*pendent and an *in*dependent variable: family change, for instance, is both affected by ageing (longer co-existence of older and younger generations gives greater scope for relationship building across generations) and affects the ageing process (a smaller family size feeds into population ageing). The fascination of ageing as an area of investigation lies in its multidimensionality and the many inter-connections between the health, economic and social aspects of ageing. Much remains to be done in researching these dimensions and their inter-connections; even more remains to be done in translating research findings into improvements in policies and practices; and the most laborious efforts remain to be undertaken in the sphere of attitudes and perceptions of ageing.

However, for a deeper and more up to date understanding of ageing societies, the readers are advised (and, having read this book, are hopefully better equipped) to observe the realities and representations of ageing in their own social contexts. Old age is not static. Its meaning changes across cultures, countries and time. Today's younger cohorts will be classified as 'older' in the future, and will in many ways extend their behaviours, preferences, expectations and lifestyles into their own old age. Who decides what the twenty-first century, the 'silver century', will look like? You and I do – we all do – as we age.

References

AARP (American Association of Retired People) (2002) *Update: A Survey of Adult Fun-Styles*. Washington, DC: AARP.

AARP (American Association of Retired People) (2007) Available at: www.aarp.org/ (accessed July 2007).

Ahern, D., Doyle, M. and Timonen, V. (2007) Regulating home care of older people: the inevitable poor relation? *Dublin University Law Journal*, 14(1).

Alber, J. (1995) A framework for the comparative study of social services, *Journal of European Social Policy*, 5(2): 131–49.

Alber, J. and Fahey, T. (2004) *Perceptions of Living Conditions in an Enlarged Europe*. Dublin: European Commission and European Foundation for the Improvement of Living and Working Conditions.

Alber, J. and Köhler, U. (2004) *Health and Care in an Enlarged Europe*. Dublin: European Commission and European Foundation for the Improvement of Living and Working Conditions.

Alber, J. and Schölkopf, M. (1999) *Senior Politics: The Social Situation of the Elderly in Germany and Europe*. Amsterdam: G+B Verlag Fakultas.

Aliaga, C. and Romans, F. (2006) The employment of seniors in the European Union, *Statistics in Focus: Population and Social Conditions*, 15/2006.

Andrews, G. R. (2001) Care of older people: promoting health and function in an ageing population, *British Medical Journal*, 322: 728–9.

Andreyeva, T., Sturm, R. and Ringel, J. S. (2004) Moderate and severe obesity have large differences in healthcare costs, *Obesity Research*, 2: 1936–43.

Antonucci, T. C. and Akiyama, H. (1987) Social relations in adult life, *Journal of Gerontology*, 4: 517–27.

Anttonen, A. and Sipilä, J. (1996) European social care services: is it possible to identify models, *Journal of European Social Policy*, 6(2): 87–100.

Anttonen, A., Baldock, J. and Sipilä, J. (eds) (2003) *The Young, the Old and the State: Social Care Systems in Five Industrial Nations*. Cheltenham: Edward Elgar.

Anttonen, A., Sipilä, J. and Baldock, J. (2003) Patterns of social care in five industrial societies: explaining diversity, in A. Anttonen, J. Baldock and J. Sipilä (eds) *The Young, the Old and the State: Social Care Systems in Five Industrial Nations*. Cheltenham: Edward Elgar.

Arber, S., Davidson, K. and Ginn, J. (eds) (2003) *Gender and Ageing: Changing Roles and Relationships*. Maidenhead: Open University Press.

Aust, A. and Bönker, F. (2004) New risks in a conservative welfare state: the case of

Germany, in P. Taylor-Gooby (ed.) *New Risk New Welfare: The Transformation of the European Welfare State*. Oxford: Oxford University Press.

Banks, J., Breeze, E., Lessof, C. and Nazroo, J. (eds) (2006) *Retirement, Health and Relationships of the Older Population in England: The 2004 English Longitudinal Study of Ageing ELSA (Wave 2)*. London: The Institute for Fiscal Studies.

Barberger-Gateau, P., Rainville, C., Letenneur, L., Dartigues, J. F. (2000) A hierarchical model of domains of disablement in the elderly: a longitudinal approach, *Disability and Rehabilitation*, 22(7): 308–17.

Begley, E. and Cahill, S. (2003) Carers: why women? *Studies*, 92(366): 162–70.

Béland, F. and Zunzunegui, M. V. (1995a) Presentación del estudio 'Envejecer en Leganés', *Revista de Gerontologia*, 5: 207–14.

Béland, F. and Zunzunegui, M. V. (1995b) El perfil de las incapacidades funcionales, *Revista de Gerontologia*, 5: 232–4.

Bengtson, V. L., Schaie, K. W. and Burton, L. (eds) (1995) *Adult Intergenerational Relations: Effects of Societal Change*. New York: Springer.

Berkman, L. F. and Kawachi, I. (eds) (2000) *Social Epidemiology*. New York: Oxford University Press.

Bernard, M., Phillips, J., Machin, L. and Harding Davies, V. (eds) (2000) *Women Ageing: Changing Identities, Challenging Myths*. London: Routledge.

Biggs, S. (1999) *The Mature Imagination: Dynamics of Identity in Midlife and Beyond*. Buckingham: Open University Press.

Bishop, C. E. (1999) Where are the missing elders? The decline in nursing home use, 1985 and 1995, *Health Affairs*, 18(4): 146–55.

Blake, D. (1995) *Pension Schemes and Pension Funds in the United Kingdom*. Oxford: Clarendon Press.

Bond, J. and Corner, L. (2004) *Quality of Life and Older People*. Buckingham: Open University Press.

Bonneux, L., Barendregt, J. J., Nusselder, W. J. and Van der Maas, P. J. (1998) Preventing fatal diseases increases healthcare costs: cause elimination life table approach, *British Medical Journal*, 316: 26–9.

Borell, K. and Ghazanfareeor Karlsson, S. (2003) "Reconceptualizing Intimacy and Ageing: Living Apart Together." In: Arber, Sara, Davidson, Kate and Ginn, Jay (Eds.) *Gender and Ageing. Changing Roles and Relationships*. Maidenhead: Open University Press.

Bowling, A. (2005) *Ageing Well: Quality of Life in Old Age*. Maidenhead: Open University Press.

Brady, D. (2003) The politics of poverty: left political institutions, the welfare state and poverty, *Social Forces*, 82(2): 557–88.

Brady, D. (2004) Reconsidering the divergence between elderly, child and overall poverty, *Research on Aging*, 26(5): 487–510.

Branch, L. G., Guralnik, J. M., Foley, D. J. et al. (1991) Active life expectancy for 10,000 Caucasian men and women in three communities, *Journals of Gerontology Series B Psychological Social Sciences*, 46(4): M145–50.

Brønnum-Hansen, H. (2005) Health expectancy in Denmark, 1987–2000, *European Journal of Public Health*, 15(1): 20–5.

Brooks, C. and Brady, D. (1999) Income, economic voting and long-term political change, 1952–1996, *Social Forces*, 77(4): 1339–75.

Brown, R. L. and Prus, S. G. (2003) Social transfers and income inequality in old age: a multi-national perspective. Luxembourg Income Study Working Paper No. 355.

Busse, R., Krauth, C. and Schwartz, F. W. (2002) Use of acute hospital beds does not increase as the population ages: results from a seven year cohort study in Germany, *Journal of Epidemiology and Community Health*, 56: 289–93.

Bytheway, B. (1994) *Ageism*. Buckingham: Open University Press.

Bytheway, B., Ward, R., Holland, C. and Peace, S. (2007) The road to an age-inclusive society, in M. Bernard and T. Scharf (eds) *Critical Perspective on Ageing Societies*. Bristol: The Policy Press.

Castles, F. G. (2003) The world turned upside down: below replacement fertility, changing preferences and family-friendly public policy in 21 OECD countries, *Journal of European Social Policy*, 13(3): 209–27.

Cavanaugh, J. C. and Whitbourne, S. K. (eds) (1999) *Gerontology: An Interdisciplinary Perspective*. New York: Oxford University Press.

Chambers, C. V., Diamond, J. J., Perkel, R. L. and Lasch, L. A. (1994) Relationship of advanced directives to hospital charges in a Medicare population, *Archives of Internal Medicine*, 154: 541–7.

Cooper, C. and Hagan, P. (1999) The ageing Australian population and future healthcare costs, 1996–2051, Occasional Papers New Series No. 7, Commonwealth Department of Health and Aged Care, Canberra.

Costa, D. L. (1998) *The Evolution of Retirement: An American Economic History, 1880–1990*. Chicago: University of Chicago Press.

Cowgill, D. O. and Holmes, L. D. (1972) *Aging and Modernisation*. New York: Appleton.

Cox, C. B. (ed.) (2000) *To Grandmother's House We Go and Stay: Perspectives on Custodial Grandparents*. New York: Springer.

Crimmins, E. (2007) Discussion On: Is the Compression of Morbidity a Worldwide Phenomenon? At the 60th Annual Scientific Meeting of the Gerontological Society of America, San Francisco, Nov. 19th, 2007.

Crimmins, E. M. (2004) Trends in the health of the elderly, *Annual Review of Public Health*, 25: 79–98.

Crimmins, E. M. and Cambois, E. (2003) Social inequalities in health expectancy, in J. M. Robine, C. Jagger, C. D. Mathers et al. (eds) *Determining Health Expectancies*. Chichester: Wiley.

Crimmins, E. M. and Saito, Y. (2000) Change in the prevalence of diseases among older Americans: 1984–94, *Demographic Research*, 3(9).

Crimmins, E. M. and Saito, Y. (2001) Trends in life expectancy in the United States, 1970–1990: gender, racial and educational differences, *Social Science and Medicine*, 52: 1629–41.

Crimmins, E. M., Hayward, M. D. and Saito, Y. (1996) Differentials in active life expectancy in the older population of the United States, *Journals of Gerontology Series B Psychological Social Sciences*, 51: S111–120.

Cullen, K., Delaney, S. and Duff, P. (2004) *Caring, Working and Public Policy*. Dublin: The Equality Authority.

Cumming, E. and Henry, W. E. (1961) *Growing Old: The Process of Disengagement*. New York: Basic Books.

Cutler, D. (2001) Declining disability among the elderly, *Health Affairs*, 20: 11–27.

Daly, M. (ed.) (2001) *Care Work: The Quest for Security*. Geneva: International Labour Office.

Daviglus, M. L., Liu, K., Pirzada, A. et al. (2003) Favourable cardiovascular risk profile in middle age and health-related quality of life in older age, *Archives of Internal Medicine*, 163: 2460–8.

Daviglus, M. L., Liu, K., Pirzada, A. et al. (2005) Cardiovascular risk profile earlier in life and Medicare costs in the last year of life, *Archives of Internal Medicine*, 165: 1028–34.

Deeg, D. J. H., Portrait, F. and Lindeboom, M. (2002) Health profiles and profile-specific health expectancies of older women and men: the Netherlands, *Journal of Women and Aging*, 14(1–2): 27–46.

Deeg, D. J. H., Tilburg, T., Smit, J. H. and de Leeuw, E. D. (2002) Attrition in the Longitudinal Ageing Study Amsterdam: the effect of differential inclusion in side studies, *Journal of Clinical Epidemiology*, 55: 319–28.

Department of Health (UK) (1990) National Health Service and Community Care Act 1990 (c. 19). Available at: www.opsi.gov.uk/ACTS/acts1990/Ukpga_19900019_en_1.htm

Department of Health (UK) (2001a) Care Standards Act 2000: guidance to local authority and health authority registration and inspection units on the transfer of registration for existing regulated providers to the National Care Standards Commission, HSC 2001/021, Department of Health (UK), London.

Department of Health (UK) (2001b) *National Service Framework For Older People: Modern Standards and Service Models*. London: HMSO.

Department of Social and Family Affairs (2002) *Study to Examine the Future Financing of Long-Term Care in Ireland*. Dublin: The Stationery Office.

Deutsche Bank Research (2002) *The Demographic Challenge: Demography Special*. Frankfurt: Deutsche Bank AG, DB Research.

DFID (Department for International Development) (2005) *Reducing Poverty by Tackling Social Exclusion: A DFID Policy Paper*. London: DFID.

Dimmock, B., Bornat, J., Peace, S. and Jones, D. (2004) Intergenerational relationships among stepfamilies in the UK, in S. Harper (ed.) *Families in Ageing Societies: A Multi-Disciplinary Approach*. Oxford: Oxford University Press.

Disney, Richard (1998) *Can We Afford To Grow Older?* Cambridge (MA) and London: MIT Press.

Dixon, T., Shaw, M., Frankel, S. and Ebrahim, S. (2004) Hospital admissions, age, and death: retrospective cohort study, *British Medical Journal*, 328: 1288.

Doblhammer, G. and Kytir, J. (1998) Social inequalities in disability-free and healthy life expectancy in Austria, *Wiener Klinische Wochenschrift*, 110: 393–6.

Doyle, M. and Timonen, V. (2007) *Home Care for Ageing Populations: A Comparative Analysis of Domiciliary Care in Denmark, Germany and the United States*. Cheltenham: Edward Elgar.

Edmonds, E., Mammen, K. and Miller, D. L. (2004) Rearranging the family? Income support and elderly living arrangements in a low income country, NBER Working Paper 10306, National Bureau of Economic Research, Massachusetts.

Emanuel, E. J. and Emanuel, L. L. (1994) The economics of dying – the illusion of cost savings at the end of life, *New England Journal of Medicine*, 330: 540–44.

Emanuel, E. J., Ash, A., Yu, W. et al. (2002) Managed care, hospice use, site of death and medical expenditures in the last year of life, *Archives of Internal Medicine*, 162: 1722–8.

Esping-Andersen, G. (1990) *The Three Worlds of Welfare Capitalism*. Princeton: Princeton University Press.

Esping-Anderson, G. (1999) *Social Foundations of Post-Industrial Economies*. Oxford: Oxford University Press.

Estes, C. (1979) *The Aging Enterprise*. San Francisco: Jossey Bass.

EC (European Commission) (2003) *European Social Statistics: Labour Force Survey Results 2002. Data 2002*. Luxembourg: Office for official Publications of the European Communities. Available at: http://epp.eurostat.ec.europa.eu/cache/ITY_OFFPUB/KS-BP-03-001/EN/KS-BP-03-001-EN.PDF

EC (European Commission) (2005) *The European Employment Strategy: A Key Component of the Lisbon Strategy*. Luxembourg: Employment and Social Affairs, EC. Available at: http://ec.europa.eu/employment_social/employment_strategy/index_en.htm#

Evandrou, M. and Glaser, K. (2003) Combining work and family life: the pension penalty of caring, *Ageing and Society*, 23(5): 583–602.

Evans, L. and Williamson, J. B. (1984) Social control of the elderly, in M. Minkler and C. L. Estes (eds) *Readings in the Political Economy of Aging. Farmingdate*. New York: Baywood Publishing.

Fahey, T. and FitzGerald, J. (1997) *Welfare Implications of Demographic Trends*. Dublin: Combat Poverty Agency.

Fahey, T., FitzGerald, J. D. and Maitre, B. (1998) The economic and social implications of demographic change, *Journal of the Statistical and Social Inquiry Society of Ireland*, 27(5).

Fine, Michael D. (2007) *A Caring Society? Care and the Dilemmas of Human Service in the 21st Century*. Basingstoke & New York: Palgrave Macmillan.

Flegal, K. M., Carroll, M. D., Kuczmarski, R. J. and Johnson, C. L. (1998) Overweight and obesity in the United States: prevalence and trends, 1960–1994, *International Journal of Obesity and Related Metabolic Disorders*, 22: 39–47.

Flegal, K. M., Carroll, M. D., Ogden, C. L. and Johnson, C. L. (2002) Prevalence and trends in obesity among US adults, *Journal of the American Medical Association*, 288: 1723–7.

Foerster, M. and Mira d'Ercole, M. (2005) Income distribution and poverty in OECD countries in the second half of the 1990s, OECD Social, Employment and Migration Working Papers No. 22.

Fortuny, M. A. and Behrendt, C. (2002) *Policy Brief on Employment and Social Protection Indicators*. Geneva: International Labour Office.

Freedman, V. A., Martin, L. G. and Schoeni, R. F. (2002) Recent trends in disability and functioning among older adults in the United States: a systematic review, *Journal of the American Medical Association*, 288: 3137–46.

Fries, J. (2003) Measuring and monitoring success in compressing morbidity, *Annals of Internal Medicine*, 139: 455–9.

Fries, J., Koop, C., Beadle, C. et al. (1993) Reducing healthcare costs by reducing the need and demand for medical services, *New England Journal of Medicine*, 329: 321–5.

Fuchs, V. R. (1984) 'Though much is taken': reflections on aging, health and medical care, *Milbank Memorial Fund quarterly: Health and society*, 62: 143–66.

Garavan, R., McGee, R. and Winder, R. (2001) *Health and Social Services for Older People (HeSSOP) Report No. 64*. Dublin: National Council for Ageing and Older People (NCAOP).

Gee, E. M. and Gutman, G. M. (2000) *The Overselling of Population Aging: Apocalyptic Demography, Intergenerational Challenges, and Social Policy*. Oxford: Oxford University Press.

Glendinning, C. (2006) Paying family care givers: evaluating different models, in C. Glendinning and P. A. Kemp (eds) *Cash and Care: Policy Challenges in the Welfare State*. Bristol: Policy Press.

Glendinning, C., Davies, B., Pickard, L. and Comas-Herrera, A. (2004) *Funding for Long-Term Care for Older People: Lessons from Other Countries*. York: Joseph Rowntree Foundation.

Gornick, M., McMillan, A. and Lubitz, J. A. (1993) A longitudinal perspective on patterns of Medicare payments, *Health Affairs*, 12(2): 140–50.

Graham, P., Blakely, T., Davis, P. et al. (2004) Compression, expansion or dynamic equilibrium? The evolution of health expectancy in New Zealand, *Journal of Epidemiology and Community Health*, 58: 659–66.

Gruber, J. and Wise, D. A. (2002) An international perspective on policies for an aging society, in S. Altman and D. Shactman (eds) *Policies for an Aging Society*. Baltimore: The Johns Hopkins Press.

Gruenberg, E. M. (1977) The failures of success, *Milbank Memorial Fund quarterly: Health and Society*, 55: 3–24.

Grundy, E. (1999) Household and family change in mid- and later life in England and Wales, in S. McRae (ed.) *Changing Britain: Families and households in the 1990s*. Oxford: Oxford University Press.

Grundy, E., Murphy, M. and Shelton, N. (1999) Looking beyond the household: intergenerational perspectives on living kin and contacts with kin in Great Britain, *Population Trends*, 97: 19–27.

Guralnik, J. M., Land, K. C., Blazer, D., Filenbaum, G. G. and Branch, L. G. (1993) Educational status and active life expectancy among older blacks and whites, *New England Journal of Medicine*, 329: 110–16.

Gutiérrez-Fisac, J. L., Gispert, R. and Sola, J. (2000) Factors explaining the geographical differences in disability free life expectancy in Spain, *Journal of Epidemiology and Community Health*, 54: 451–55.

Hamel, M. B., Phillips, R. S., Teno, J. M. et al. (1996) Seriously ill hospitalized adults: do we spend less on older patients? *Journal of the American Geriatrics Society*, 44: 1043–8.

Hamel, M. B., Teno, J. M., Goldman, L. et al. (1999) Patient age and decisions to withhold life-sustaining treatments from seriously ill hospitalized adults, *Annals of Internal Medicine*, 130: 116–25.

Hamel, M. B., Lynn, J., Teno, J. M. et al. (2000) Age-related differences in care preferences, treatment decisions and clinical outcomes in seriously ill hospitalised adults: lessons from SUPPORT, *Journal of the American Geriatrics Society*, 48: S176–82.

Harper, S. (ed.) (2004) *Families in Ageing Societies: A Multi-Disciplinary Approach*. Oxford: Oxford University Press.

Harper, S. (2006) *Ageing Societies: Myths, Challenges and Opportunities*. New York: Hodder Arnold.

Hellerstein, J., Neumark, D. and Troske, K. (1999) Wages, productivity and worker characteristics. Evidence from plant level production functions and wage equations, *Journal of Labor Economics*, 17(3): 409–46.

Henretta, J. C., Hill, M. S., Li, W., Soldo, B. J. and Wolf, D. A. (1997) Selection of children to provide care: the effect of earlier parental transfers, *Journal of Gerontology Series B: Psychological Sciences and Social Sciences*, 52B: 110–19.

Hermalin, A. I., Roan, C. and Perez, A. (1998) The emerging role of grandparents in Asia: Comparative study of the elderly in Asia, Research report No 98, Population Studies Centre University of Michigan, Ann Arbor.

Hiraoka, K. (2004) Long-Term care Insurance in Japan, in Y. Hyunsook and J. Hendricks (eds) *Handbook of Asian Ageing*. New York: Baywood Publishing.

Hobson, B. (1990) No exit, no voice: women's economic dependency and the welfare state, *Acta Sociologica*, 33(3): 235–50.

Hoff, A. (2007) Patterns of Intergenerational Support in Grandparent-Grandchild and Parent-Child Relationships in Germany. *Ageing and Society* Vol. 27(5): 643–65.

Hogan, C., Lunney, J., Gabel, J. et al. (2001) Medicare beneficiaries' costs of care in the last year of life, *Health Affairs (Millwood)*, 20: 188–95.

Hubert, H. B., Bloch, D. A., Oehlert, J. W. et al. (2002) Lifestyle habits and compression of morbidity, *Journals of Gerontology Series A: Biological Sciences and Medical Sciences*, 57A: M 347–51.

Huebschmann, A. D. G., Bublitz, C. and Anderson, R. J. (2006) Are hypertensive elderly patients treated differently? *Clinical Interventions in Aging*, 3(1): 289–94.

Hughes, M. E. and Waite, L. J. (2004) The American family as a context for healthy ageing, in S. Harper (ed.) *Families in Ageing Societies: A Multi-Disciplinary Approach*. Oxford: Oxford University Press.

Hughes, G., Williams, J. and Blackwell, S. (2005) Demand and cost of long-term care services, Country Report for the GALCA project (Ireland), Economic and Social Research Institute, Dublin.

Jacobzone, S. (1999) *Ageing and Care for Frail Elderly Persons: An Overview of International Perspectives*. Paris: Organisation for Economic Co-operation and Development.

Jacobzone, S. (2000) Health and ageing: international perspectives on long term care, *Isuma Canadian Journal of Policy Research*, 1(2). Available at: www.isuma.net/v01n02/jacobzone/jacobzone_e.shtml

Janssen, F., Mackenbach, J. P. and Kunst, A. E. (2004) NEDCOM. Trends in old-age mortality in seven European countries, 1950–1999, *Journal of Clinical Epidemiology*, 57: 203–16.

Jitapunkul, S., Kunanusont, C., Phoolcharoen, W. et al. (2003) Disability-free life expectancy of elderly people in a population undergoing demographic and epidemiologic transition, *Age Ageing*, 32: 401–5.

Johnson, M. F. and Kramer, A. M. (2000) Physicians' responses to clinical scenarios involving life-threatening illness vary by patients' age, *Journal of Clinical Ethics*, 11: 323–7.

Johnson, R. W. and Lo Sasso, A. T. (2004) Family support of the elderly and female labour supply: trade-offs among care giving, financial transfers and work: evidence from the HRS, in S. Harper (ed.) *Families in Ageing Societies: A Multi-Disciplinary Approach*. Oxford: Oxford University Press.

Jylhä, M., Jokela, J., Tolvanen, E. et al. (1992) The Tampere Longitudinal Study on Ageing, description of the study, basic results on health and functional ability, *Scandinavian Journal of Social Medicine: Supplementum*, 47: 1–4.

Kamiya, Y. (2006) Social security and living arrangements of the elderly in Brazil, unpublished PhD thesis, University of California, Berkeley.

Kangas, O. and Palme, J. (1998) Does social policy matter? Poverty cycles in OECD countries, Luxembourg Income Study Working Paper No. 187.

Kapteyn, A. and De Vos, K. (1998) Social security and labor force participation in the Netherlands, *American Economic Review*, 88(2): 164–7.

Katz, S., Downs, T. D., Cash, H. R. et al. (1970) Progress in development of the index of ADL, *Gerontologist*, 10: 20–30.

Katz, S., Branch, L. G. and Branson, M. H. (1983) Active life expectancy, *New England Journal of Medicine*, 309: 1218–24.

Kautto, M. (2002) Investing in Services in West European welfare states, *Journal of European Social Policy*, 12: 55.

Kemper, P. and Murtaugh, C. M. (1991) Lifetime use of nursing home care, *New England Journal of Medicine*, 324: 595–600.

Kinsella, K. G. and Velkoff, V. A. (2001) *An Aging World*. Washington: US Department of Commerce, Economics and Statistics Administration.

Kohl, J. (1981) Trends and problems in post-war public expenditure development in Western Europe and North America, in P. Flora and A. J. Heidenheimer (eds) *The Development of Welfare States in Europe and America*. New Brunswick, NJ: Transaction Books.

Kreager, P. and Schroeder-Butterfill, E. (eds) (2005) *Ageing Without Children: European and Asian Perspectives on Elderly Access to Support Networks*. Oxford and New York: Berghahn Books.

Kunst, A. E., Groenhof, F., Mackenbach, J. P. and the EU Working Group on Socioeconomic Inequalities in Health (1998) Occupational class and cause-specific mortality in middle-aged men in 11 European countries: comparison of population-based studies, *British Medical Journal*, 316: 1636–42.

Lakdawalla, D. N., Bhattacharya, J. and Goldman, D. P. (2004) Are the young becoming more disabled? *Health Affairs*, 23: 168–76.

Lansley, P., McCreadie, C., Tinker, A. et al. (2004) Adapting the homes of older people: a case study of costs and savings, *Building Research and Information*, 32(6): 468–83.

Laslett, P. (1996) *A Fresh Map of Life: The Emergence of the Third Age*. Basingstoke and London: McMillan.

Lawton, M. P. and Brody, E. M. (1969) Assessment of older people: self-maintaining and instrumental activities of daily living, *Gerontologist*, 9: 179–86.

Leeson, G. W. (2004) The demographics and economics of UK health and social care for older adults, Working Paper WP 304, Oxford Institute of Ageing, Oxford.

Levinsky, N. G., Ash, A. S., Yu, W. and Moskowitz, M. A. (1999) Patterns of use of major procedures in medical care of older adults, *Journal of the American Geriatrics Society*, 47: 553–8.

Levinsky, N. G., Yu, W., Ash, A. et al. (2001) Influence of age on Medicare expenditures and medical care in the last year of life, *Journal of American Medical Association*, 286(11): 1349–55.

Lewis, J. (1992) Gender and the development of welfare regimes, *Journal of European Social Policy*, 2(3): 159–73.

Loughran, D. S. and Seabury, S. A. (2007) *Estimating the Accident Risk of Older Drivers*. Santa Monica: RAND.

Lubitz, J. and Prihoda, R. (1984) The use and costs of Medicare services in the last two years of life, *Health Care Financial Review*, 5: 117–31.

Lubitz, J. and Riley, G. F. (1993) Trends in Medicare payments in the last year of life, *New England Journal Medicine*, 328: 1092–6.

Lubitz, J., Beebe, J. and Baker, C. (1995) Longevity and medicare expenditures, *New England Journal Medicine*, 332: 999–1003.

Luce, J. M. and Rubenfeld, G. D. (2002) Can health care costs be reduced by limiting intensive care at the end of life? *American Journal of Respiratory and Critical Care Medicine*, 165: 750–4.

Lundsgaard, J. (2005) *Consumer Direction and Choice in Long-Term Care for Older Persons, Including Payments for Informal Care: How Can it Help Improve Care Outcomes, Employment and Fiscal Sustainability?* Paris: OECD.

Maggi, S., Zucchetto, M., Grigoletto, F. et al. (1994) The Italian Longitudinal Study on Ageing (ILSA): design and methods, *Aging Clinical and Experimental Research*, 6: 464–73.

Maksoud, A., Jahnigen, D. W. and Skibinski, C. I. (1993) Do not resuscitate orders and the cost of death, *Archives of Internal Medicine*, 153: 1249–53.

Mandin, C. and Palier, B. (2003) Policy maps: France, Working Paper (WRAMSOC project), University of Kent, Kent.

Manton, K. G. (1982) Changing concepts of morbidity and mortality in the elderly population, *Milbank Memorial Fund Quarterly: Health and Society*, 60: 183–244.

Manton, K. G and Gu, X. (2001) Changes in the prevalence of chronic disability in the United States black and non-black population above 65 from 1982 to 1999, *Proceedings of the National Academy of Science of the United States of America*, 98: 6354–9.

Manton, K. G. and Land, K. C. (2000) Active life expectancy estimates for the United States elderly population: a multidimensional continuous-mixture model of functional change applied to completed cohorts, 1982–1996, *Demography*, 37(3): 253–65.

Manton, K. G., Corder, L. and Stallard, E. (1997) Chronic disability trends in elderly United States populations 1982–94, *Proceedings of the National Academy of Science of the United States of America*, 94: 2593–8.

Manton, K. G., Stallard, E. and Corder, L. (1997) Changes in the age dependence of mortality and disability: cohort and other determinants, *Demography*, 34: 135–57.

Manza, J. and Brooks, C. (1999) *Social Cleavages and Political Change: Voter Alignments and U.S. Party Coalitions*. New York: Oxford University Press.

Marmor, T., Fay, R., Cook, L. and Scher, S. (1997) Social security and the conflict between generations: are we asking the right questions? in E. R. Kingson and J. H. Schulz (eds) *Social Security in the 21st Century*. New York: Oxford University Press.

Marmot, M., Banks, J., Blundell, R., Lessof, C. and Nazroo, J. (2003) *Health, Wealth and Lifestyles of the Older Population in England: The 2002 English Longitudinal Study of Ageing*. London: Institute of Fiscal Studies.

Marmot, Michael and Wilkinson, Richard G. (2006) (Eds.) *Social Determinants of Health*. Oxford: Oxford University Press.

Mathers, C. D., Sadana, R., Salomon, J. A., Murray, C. J. and Lopez, A. D. (2001) Healthy life expectancy in 191 countries, 1999, *Lancet*, 357: 1685–91.

May, J., Govender, J., Budlender, D. et al. (1998) Poverty and inequality in South Africa, Report prepared for the Office of the Executive Deputy

President and the inter-ministerial committee for poverty and inequality, Praxis, Durban.

McGivern, Y. (ed.) (2001) *Employment and Retirement Among the Over-55s: Patterns, Preferences and Issues*. Dublin: National Council on Ageing and Older People.

Minicuci, N. and Noale, M. (2005) Disability-free life expectancy in older Italians, *Disability and Rehabilitation*, 27(5): 221–7.

Minicuci, N., Noale, M., Bardage, C. et al. (2003) Cross-national determinants of quality of life from six longitudinal studies on aging: the CLESA project, *Aging Clinical and Experimental Research*, 15: 187–202.

Minicuci, N., Noale, M., Pluijm, S. et al. (2004) Disability-free life expectancy: a cross-national comparison of six longitudinal studies on ageing: the CLESA project, *European Journal of Ageing*, 1(1): 37–44.

Mor, V. (2005) The compression of morbidity hypothesis: a review of research and prospects for the future, *Journal of the American Geriatrics Society*, 53(9): S308–311.

Morel, N. (2006) Providing coverage against new social risks in Bismarckian welfare states: the case of long term care, in K. Armingeon and G. Bonoli (eds) *The Politics of Postindustrial Welfare States: Adapting Postwar Social Polices to New Social Risks*. London: Routledge.

Moreno, L. (2004) Spain's transition to new welfare: a farewell to superwomen, in P. Taylor-Gooby (ed.) *New Risks, New Welfare: The Transformation of the European Welfare*. Oxford: Oxford University Press.

Motel-Klingebiel, A., Tesch-Roemer, C. and von Kondratowitz, H. (2005) Welfare states do not crowd out the family: evidence for mixed responsibility from comparative analyses, *Ageing and Society*, 25(6): 863–82.

Mujahid, G. (2006) Population ageing in East and South-East Asia, 1950–2050: implications for elderly care, *Asia-Pacific Population Journal*, 21(2).

Myles, J. (2002) A New contract for the elderly? in G. Esping-Andersen, D. Gallie, A. Hemerijk and J. Myles (eds) *Why We Need a New Welfare State*. Oxford: Oxford University Press.

Myles, J. (2003) What justice requires: pension reform in ageing societies, *Journal of European Social Policy*, 13(3): 264–9.

Myles, J. and Pierson, P. (2001) The comparative political economy of pension reform, in P. Pierson (ed.) *The New Politics of the Welfare State*. Oxford: Oxford University Press.

National Statistics UK (2007) Available at: www.statistics.gov.uk/CCI/SearchRes.asp?term=expectancy

NCAOP (National Council for Ageing and Older People) (2005) *Health and Social Services for Older People II (HeSSOP II). Changing Profiles from 2000 to 2004*. Dublin: NCAOP.

Netten, A., Williams, J. and Darton, R. (2005) Care-home closures in England: causes and implications, *Ageing and Society*, 25(3).

OECD (1996) *Ageing in OECD Countries: A Critical Policy Challenge*. Paris: OECD.

OECD (2004) *Dementia Care in Nine OECD Countries. A Comparative Analysis*. Paris: OECD.

OECD (2005) *Long-Term Care Policies for Older People*. Paris: OECD.

OECD (2007) *Pensions at a Glance*. Available at: www.oecd.org/document/35/ 0,3343,en_2649_201185_38717411_1_1_1_1,00.html

Oeppen, J. and Vaupel, J. W. (2002) Broken limits to life expectancy, *Science*, 296: 1029–31.

Ogg, J. and Renaut, S. (2006) The support of parents in old age by those born during 1945–1954: a European perspective, *Ageing and Society*, 26(5): 723–43.

Oppong, C. (2006) Familial roles and social transformations: older men and women in Sub-Saharan Africa, *Research on Aging*, 28(6): 654–68.

Orloff, A. S. (1993) Gender and the social rights of citizenship: the comparative analysis of gender relations and welfare states, *American Sociological Review*, 58(3): 303–28.

Pampel, F. (1994) Population aging, class context and age inequality in public spending, *American Journal of Sociology*, 100: 153–95.

Patsios, D. (2000) Poverty and social exclusion amongst the elderly, Working Paper No. 20, Poverty and Social Exclusion Survey of Britain, Townsend Centre for International Poverty Research.

Peace, S. M., Kellaher, L. and Willcocks, D. (1997) *Re-Evaluating Residential Care*. Buckingham: Open University Press.

Pebley, A. R. (1998) Demography and the environment, *Demography*, 35(4): 377–89.

Pedersen, N. L. (1991) The Swedish Adoption Twin Study of Aging: an update, *Acta Geneticae Medicae et Gemellologiae (Roma)*, 40: 7–20.

Peeters, A., Barendregt, J. J., Willekens, F. et al. (2003) Obesity in adulthood and its consequences for life expectancy: a life-table analysis, *Annals of Internal Medicine*, 138: 24–32.

Perenboom, R. J., Van Herten, L. M., Boshuizen, H. C. and Van Den Bos, G. A. (2004) Trends in disability-free life expectancy, *Disability and Rehabilitation*, 26: 377–86.

Pérès, K., Jagger, C., Lievre, A. and Barberger-Gateau, P. (2005) Disability-free life expectancy of older French people: gender and education differentials from the PAQUID cohort, *European Journal of Ageing*, 2(3): 225–33.

Phillips, J., Bernard, M. and Chittenden, M. (2002) *Juggling Work and Care: The Experience of Working Carers of Older Adults*. Bristol: Policy Press.

Phillipson, C. (1982) *Capitalism and the Construction of Old Age*. London: Macmillan.

Phillipson, C., Bernard, M., Phillips, J. and Ogg, J. (2001) *The Family and Community Life of Old People*. London: Routledge.

Pickard, L., Wittenberg, R., Comas-Herrera, A., Davies, B. and Darton, R. (2000) Relying on informal care in the new century? Informal care for elderly people in England to 2031, *Ageing and Society*, 20: 745–72.

Preston, S. H. (1984) Children and the elderly: divergent paths for America's dependents, *Demography*, 21: 435–57.

Project OASIS Expert Committee (1999) *First Report of Project OASIS* (Old Age Social and Income Security). Available at: www.seniorindian.com/oasis__.htm

Quinn, J. F. (1999) Has the early retirement trend reversed? Working Papers in Economics 424. Boston College Department of Economics, Boston.

Quinn, J. F., Burkhauser, R., Cahill, K. and Weather, R. (1998) Microeconometric analysis of the retirement decision (in the United States), Economics Department Working Paper No. 203, OECD, Paris.

Qureshi, H. and Walker, A. (1998) *The Caring Relationship*. London: Macmillan.

Raju, S. (2004) Economic issue of elderly in India, *Harmony Magazine*.

RAND Europe (2005) *Population Implosion? Low Fertility and Policy Responses in the European Union*, Research Brief. Cambridge: RAND.

Robine, J. M., Romieu, I. and Cambois, E. (1999) Health expectancy indicators, *Bulletin of the World Health Organization*, 77: 181–5.

Robine, J. M., Jagger, C. and Cambois, E. (2002) European perspectives on healthy aging in women, *Journal of Women and Aging*, 14: 119–33.

Roos, N. P., Montgomery, P. and Roos, L. L. (1987) Health care utilization in the years prior to death, *The Millbank Quarterly*, 65: 231–54.

Rosenmayr, L. (1977) The family: a source of hope for the elderly, in E. Shanas, and M. B. Sussman, (eds) *Family, Bureaucracy, and the Elderly*. Durham, NC: Duke University.

Rosow, I. and Breslau, N. (1966) A Guttman health scale for the aged, *Journal of Gerontology B Psychological Sciences and Social Science*, 21: 556–9.

Rowe, J. W. and Kahn, R. L. (1999) *Successful Aging*. New York: Pantheon Random House.

Rowntree, S. (1901) *Poverty: A Study of Town Life*. London: McMillan.

Royal Commission (1999) With respect to old age – long-term care: rights and responsibilities, CM 4192-II, HMSO, London.

Ruspini, E. (1998) Women and poverty dynamics: the case of Germany and Britain, *Journal of European Social Policy*, 8(4): 291–316.

Sainsbury, D. (ed.) (1994) *Gendering Welfare States*. London: Sage.

Scharf, T. and Wenger, C. G. (eds) (1995) *International Perspectives on Community Care for Older People*. Avebury: Aldershot.

Scharlach, Andrew (2007) Home Care Policies in the United States. Paper presented at Trinity College Dublin, 12 March 2007.

Schroeder-Butterfill, E. (2003) Pillars of the family – support provided by the elderly in Indonesia, Working Paper No. 303, Oxford Institute of Ageing, Oxford.

Seeman, T. E., Bruce, M. L. and McAvay, G. J. (1996) Social network characteristics and onset of ADL disability: MacArthur studies of successful aging, *Journal of Gerontology B Psychological Sciences and Social Science*, 51: s191–200.

Sen, A. (1994) Population: delusion and reality, *The New York Review of Books*, 41(15): 62–71.

Sheldon, J. H. (1948) *The Social Medicine of Old Age*. Oxford: Oxford University Press.

Silverstein, M., Cong, Z. and Shuzhuo, L. (2006) Intergenerational transfers and living arrangements of older people in rural China: consequences for psychological well-being, *Journal of Gerontology B Psychological Sciences and Social Science*, 61: S256–S266.

Sipilä, J., Anttonen, A. and Baldock, J. (2003) The importance of care, in A. Anttonen, J. Baldock and J. Sipilä (eds) *The Young, the Old and the State: Social Care Systems in Five Industrial Nations*. Cheltenham: Edward Elgar.

Smith, J. P. and Kington, S. (1997) Race, socio-economic status and health in later life, in L. G Martin and B. J. Sodo (eds) *Racial and Ethnic Differences in the Health of Older Americans*. Washington: National Academy Press.

Smith, J. P., Juster, F. T. and Willis, R. J. (1999) *Wealth, Work and Health: Innovations in Measurement in the Social Sciences*. Ann Arbor: University of Michigan Press.

Socialstyrelsen (2003) *Socialtjänsten i Sverige, Vård och omsorg om äldre*. Stockholm: Socialstyrelsen, ch. 9.

Sonnenfeld, J. (1986) Heroes in collision: chief executive retirement and the parade of future leaders, *Human Resource Management*, 25(2): 305–33.

Statistics Sweden (SBC) Available at www.scb.se

Steel, K. (2005) The old-old-old, *Journal American Geriatric Society*, 53: S314–16.

Stewart, J. (ed.) (2005) *For Richer, For Poorer: An Investigation of the Irish Pension System*. Dublin: TASC.

Sturm, R., Ringel, J. and Andreyeva, T. (2004) Increasing obesity rates and disability trends, *Health Affairs*, 23: 199–205.

Sundström, G and Malmberg, B. (1996) The long arm of the welfare state shortened: home help in Sweden, *International Journal of Social Welfare*, 5(2): 69–75.

Tester, S. (1996) *Community Care for Older People: A Comparative Perspective*. Oxford: MacMillan, Houndmills.

Thane, P. (1998) The family lives of older people, in P. Johnson and P. Thane (eds) *Old Age from Antiquity to Postmodernity*. London: Routledge.

Thane, P. (2000) *Old Age in English History*. Oxford: Oxford University Press.

Timonen, V. (2005) Policy paradigms and long-term care: convergence or continuing difference in P. Taylor-Gooby (ed.) *Ideas and Welfare State Reform in Western Europe*. Basingstoke: Palgrave MacMillan, pp. 30–53.

Timonen, V. (2006) Responsibility for the costs of institutional long-term care: a comparative perspective, in E. O'Dell (ed.) *Older People in Modern Ireland: Essays on Law and Policy*. Dublin: First Law, pp. 427–49.

Timonen, V., Convery, J. and Cahill, S. (2006) Care revolutions in the making? A comparison of cash-for-care programmes in four European countries, *Ageing and Society*, 26: 455–74.

Timonen, V., Doyle, M. and Prendergast, D. (2006) *No Place Like Home: Study of Domiciliary Care Services for Older People*. Dublin: Liffey Press.

Townsend, P. (1957) *The Family Life of Old People: An Inquiry in East London*. London: Routledge.

Townsend, P. (1981) The structured dependency of the elderly: the creation of social policy in the twentieth century, *Ageing and Society*, 1(1): 5–28.

Uhlenberg, P. (1993) Demographic change and kin relationships in later life, in G. Maddox and M. P. Lawton (eds) *Annual Review of Gerontology and Geriatrics*, vol. 13. New York: Springer.

Uhlenberg, P. (1995) Demographic influences on intergenerational relationships, in V. L. Bengtson, K. W. Schaie, and L. Burton, (eds) *Adult Intergenerational Relations: Effects of Societal Change*. New York: Springer.

UNAIDS, UNICEF and USAID (2004) *Children on the Brink 2004: A Joint Report of New Orphan Estimates and a Framework for Action*. New York: USAID.

Ungerson, C. (2004) Whose empowerment and independence? A cross-national perspective on 'cash for care' schemes, *Ageing and Society*, 24: 189–92.

United Nations (1999) *The Sex and Age Distribution of the World Populations: The 1998 Revision, Vol. II: Sex and Age*. Medium Variant Projections. 8. New York: Population Division of the Department of Economic and Social Affairs (DESA), United Nations Secretariat.

United Nations (2002) *World Population Ageing 1950–2050*. New York: Population Division of the Department of Economic and Social Affairs (DESA), United Nations Secretariat.

United Nations (2007a) *World Demographic Trends*, E/CN.9/2007/6. New York: Commission on Population and Development, Economic and Social Council, United Nations. Available at: http://daccessdds.un.org/doc/UNDOC/GEN/N07/206/11/PDF/N0720611.pdf?OpenElement

United Nations (2007b) *World Population Prospects* (2006 revision). New York: Population Division of the Department of Economic and Social Affairs (DESA), United Nations Secretariat.

United Nations (2007c) *World Population Ageing 2007*. New York: Population Division of the Department of Economic and Social Affairs (DESA), United Nations Secretariat.

Valderrama-Gama, E., Damian, J., Ruigomez, A. and Martin-Moreno, J. M. (2002) Chronic disease, functional status, and self-ascribed causes of disabilities among noninstitutionalised older people in Spain, *Journal of Gerontology Series A: Biological Science and Medical Science*, 57: M716–21.

Valkonen, T., Sihvonen, A. P. and Lahelma, E. (1997) Health expectancy by level of education in Finland, *Social Science and Medicine*, 44: 801–8.

Verbrugge, L. M. (1989) The twain meet: empirical explanations of sex differences in health and mortality, *Journal of Health and Social Behavior*, 30: 282–304.

Verbrugge, L. M. and Patrick, D. L. (1995) Seven chronic conditions: their impact on US adults' activity levels and use of medical services, *American Journal of Public Health*, 85: 173–82.

Victor, C. R., Scambler, S., Bond, J. and Bowling, A. (2001) Loneliness in later life: preliminary findings from the Growing Older Project, *Quality in Ageing*, 3(1): 34–41.

Victor, C. R., Scambler, S. J., Bond, J. and Bowling, A. (2004) Loneliness in later life, in A. Walker and C. Hennessey (eds) *Quality of Life in Old Age*. Maidenhead: Open University Press.

Victor, C. R., Scambler, S. J., Bowling, A. and Bond, J. (2005) The prevalence of, and risk factors for, loneliness in later life: a survey of older people in Great Britain, *Ageing and Society*, 25(3): 357–75.

Visco, I. (2001) The fiscal implications of ageing populations in OECD countries, Working Paper No. 11 (4/01), Oxford Institute of Ageing, Oxford.

Vita, A. J., Terry, R. B., Hubert, H. P. et al. (1998) Aging, health risks and cumulative disability, *New England Journal of Medicine*, 338: 1035–41.

Vladeck, B. C. (2005) Economic and policy implications of improving longevity, *Journal of the American Geriatrics Society*, 53: S304–07.

Wærness, K. (1978) The invisible welfare state: women's work at home, *Acta Sociologica*, 21: 193–207.

Walker, A. (1980) The social creation of poverty and dependency in old age, *Journal of Social Policy*, 9(1): 45–75.

Walker, A. (1981) Towards a political economy of old age, *Ageing and Society*, 1(1): 73–94.

Walker A. (1993) *Age and Attitudes: Main Results from a Eurobarometer Survey*. Brussels: Commission of the European Communities.

Walker, A. (ed.) (2005) *Understanding Quality of Life in Old Age*. Buckingham: Open University Press.

Walker, A. and Hagan Hennessy, C. (eds) (2004) *Growing Older: Quality of Life in Old Age*. New York: Open University Press.

Walker, A. and Naegele, G. (eds) (1999) *The Politics of Old Age in Europe*. Buckingham: Open University Press.

Walter-Ginzburg, A., Guralnik, J. M., Blumstein, T., Gindin, J. and Baruch, M. (2001) Assistance with personal care activities among the old-old in Israel: a national epidemiological study, *Journal of the American Geriatrics Society*, 49(9): 1176–84.

Wenger, G. C. (1984) *The Supportive Network*. London: George Allen and Unwin.

Wilson, G. (2000) *Understanding Old Age: Critical and Global Perspectives*. London: Sage Publications.

Wolf, M. (2004) Lessons from Britain's pensions dilemma, *Financial Times*, 20 August.

Wolf, D. A., Freedman, V. A. and Soldo, B. J. (1997) The division of family labor: care for elderly parents, *Journal of Gerontology Series B: Psychological Sciences and Social Sciences*, 52B: 102–9.

World Bank (1994) *Averting the Old Age Crisis*. New York: Oxford University Press.

WHO (World Health Organisation) (2002) *The World Health Report 2002: Reducing Risks, Promoting Healthy Life*. Paris: WHO.

Wrigley, E. A. and Schofield, R. S. (1989) *The Population History of England, 1541–1871*. Cambridge: Cambridge University Press.

Yan, L. L., Daviglus, M. L., Garside, D. B. et al. (2003) Favorable cardiovascular risk status in middle age and Medicare diagnoses of coronary heart disease, stroke, cardiovascular diseases and diabetes mellitus in older age, *Circulation*, 107: e7037.

Yu, W., Ash, A. S., Levinsky, N. G. and Moskowitz, M. A. (2000) Intensive care unit use and mortality in the elderly, *Journal of General Internal Medicine*, 15: 97–102.

Index

Locators shown in *italics* refer to boxes, figures and tables.

TOM KITWOOD ON DEMENTIA

A Reader and Critical Commentary

Clive Baldwin and Andrea Capstick

- How does Kitwood's work contribute to our understanding of 'the dementing process' and the essentials of quality care?

- How was Kitwood's thinking about dementia influenced by the wider context of his work in theology, psychology and biochemistry?

- What is the relevance today of key themes and issues in Kitwood's work?

Tom Kitwood was one of the most influential writers on dementia of the last 20 years. Key concepts and approaches from his work on person-centred care and well-being in dementia have gained international recognition and shaped much current thinking about practice development. The complexities of Kitwood's work and the development of his thinking over time have, however, received less attention. This Reader brings together twenty original publications by Kitwood which span the entire period of his writing on dementia, and the different audiences for whom he wrote.

Almost ten years after Kitwood's death, it is now timely to review his contribution to the field of dementia studies in the light of more recent developments and from a critical and interdisciplinary perspective. The introduction to this Reader summarises and problematises some of the key characteristics of Kitwood's writing. Each of the four themed sections begins with a commentary offering a balanced consideration of the strengths of Kitwood's work, but also of its limitations and oversights. The Reader also includes a biography and annotated bibliography.

Tom Kitwood on Dementia: A Reader and Critical Commentary is key reading for students of social work or mental health nursing, with an interest in dementia care. Professionals working with people with dementia will also find it invaluable.

Additional Contributors: *Habib Chaudhury, Deborah O'Connor, Alison Phinney, Barbara Purves, Ruth Bartlett.*

Contents: *Acknowledgements - About the Editors - Introduction - Section 1: Critique of the standard paradigm - Section 2: Ill-being, well-being and psychological need - Section 3: Personhood - Section 4: Organisational culture and its transformation - Bibliography - References.*

2007   384pp
978-0-335-22271-1 (Paperback)   978-0-335-22272-8 (Hardback)

AGING WELL

Quality of Life in Old Age

Ann Bowling

- What is quality of life?

- What is quality of life in older age?

- How can quality of life in older age be improved?

This book explores concepts of quality of life in older age in the theoretical literature and presents the views of a national sample of people aged sixty-five years or older. It offers a broad overview of the quality of life experienced by older people in Britain using a number of wide ranging indicators, including:

- Health

- Hobbies and interests

- Home and neighbourhood

- Income

- Independence

- Psychological wellbeing

- Social and family relationships

The result is a fascinating book enlivened by rich data - both quantitative and qualitative - drawn from detailed surveys and interviews with almost a thousand older people.

Ageing Well is key reading for students, academics, practitioners and policy makers who are concerned with the research and practice that will help to improve quality of life for older people.

Contents: *Preface - List of abbreviations - Models of quality of life in older age - The study: Aims, methods, measures, sample, response rates - What adds quality to life, and what takes quality away? - Social relationships and activities - Health and functioning - Psychological outlook - Social capital: Home and neighbourhood - Financial circumstances and having enough money - Independence and freedom - Life 18 months later - Discussion: Implications for ageing well in the 21st century - Glossary - References - Index.*

2005   288pp
978-0-335-21509-6 (Paperback)   978-0-335-21510-2 (Hardback)

ENVIRONMENT AND IDENTITY IN LATER LIFE

Sheila Peace, Leonie Kellaher and Caroline Holland

Throughout life, our everyday interactions with material, social, and psychological environments influence our self identity: and 'who we think we are' influences how we behave in particular places. In later life, people bring to this relationship a lifetime's experience that makes certain associations more or less important. This book explores the relationship between environment and identity for older people.

In this detailed ethnographic study, older people talk in depth about their situations and experiences of space and place. The book examines the experience of men and women of different ages and cultures living in a range of different kinds of places, including 'ordinary' and 'special' housing - from a high-rise flat to a residential care home - in semi-rural, urban and metropolitan locations within the Midlands and south-east England.

This research enables us to appreciate how older people manage their needs within the context of their whole lives. Many are able to achieve a 'life of quality' as they constantly engage and re-engage with their environment. The discussion of how environmental complexity influences people in developing and maintaining their own identity is essential for those involved in planning, designing, caring and supporting people as they age.

Environment and Identity in Later Life is key reading for students, practitioners and policy makers interested in quality of life for older people.

Contents: *List of figures and tables - Placing the self - Housing histories - Location, location, location - Thresholds - Homing in - Pacing the self - Living the layered environment - Tracing the self - References - Index.*

2005   192pp
978-0-335-21511-9 (Paperback)   978-0-335-21512-6 (Hardback)

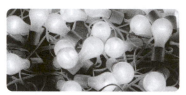
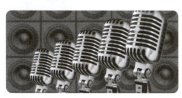
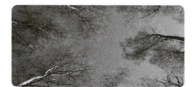
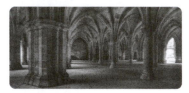
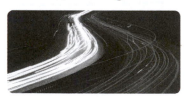
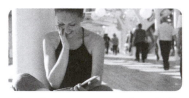
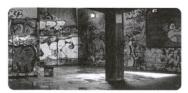